Handbook of Small Animal MRI

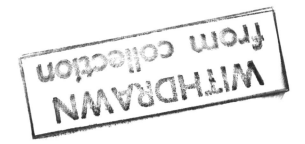

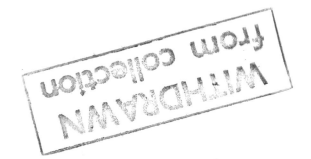

Handbook of Small Animal MRI

Ian Elliott DCR(R) DipHSW(Open)
Burgess Diagnostics Ltd, Leyland, Lancashire, UK

Geoff Skerritt FRCVS, BVSc, DECVN, CBiol, MIBiol
ChesterGates Referral Hospital, Chestergates, Chester, UK

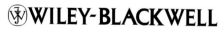

WILEY-BLACKWELL

A John Wiley & Sons, Ltd., Publication

This edition first published 2010
© Ian Elliott and Geoff Skerritt

Blackwell Publishing was acquired by John Wiley & Sons in February 2007. Blackwell's publishing programme has been merged with Wiley's global Scientific, Technical, and Medical business to form Wiley-Blackwell.

Registered office
John Wiley & Sons Ltd, The Atrium, Southern Gate, Chichester, West Sussex, PO19 8SQ, United Kingdom

Editorial office
9600 Garsington Road, Oxford, OX4 2DQ, United Kingdom
2121 State Avenue, Ames, Iowa 50014-8300, USA

For details of our global editorial offices, for customer services and for information about how to apply for permission to reuse the copyright material in this book please see our website at www.wiley.com/wiley-blackwell.

Library of Congress Cataloging-in-Publication Data
Elliott, Ian, 1954–
    Handbook of small animal MRI / Ian Elliott, Geoff Skerritt.
        p. ; cm.
    Includes bibliographical references and index.
    ISBN 978-1-4051-2650-2 (pbk. : alk. paper)
    1. Veterinary radiography–Handbooks, manuals, etc. 2. Magnetic resonance imaging–Handbooks, manuals, etc. I. Skerritt, G. C. II. Title.
        [DNLM: 1. Magnetic Resonance Imaging–instrumentation. 2. Magnetic Resonance Imaging–veterinary. 3. Safety Management. SF 757.8 E46h 2010]
    SF757.8.E45 2010
    636.089'607548–dc22
                                            2009023940

A catalogue record for this book is available from the British Library.
Set in 10/13pt Franklin Gothic Book by Toppan Best-set Premedia Limited
Printed and bound in Singapore by Ho Printing Singapore Pte Ltd

1 2010

Contents

PART ONE
Physical Principles of MRI

1 Basic Principles

At the time of writing, most veterinary professionals, whether they be surgeons, nurses or students, would probably agree that their knowledge of magnetic resonance imaging (MRI) physics borders on non-existent. Indeed, many may be filled with a deep dread at the very thought of the subject. On the other hand most will have a working knowledge of radiography at least sufficient to know that a radiograph represents a record of the different densities of body tissues through which the x-ray beam has passed. In this chapter the nature of magnetic resonance (MR) will be examined and the measurement parameters involved in constructing a MR image will be discussed.

It is worth beginning by recapping briefly on some radiation physics. In conventional radiography and computed tomography (CT), image contrast, or greyscale, is dependent on density or, more specifically, electron density of tissues in the patient. The more electrons an atom has in its shell the more it will attenuate the x-ray beam. Dense tissues, such as cortical bone, will appear as white in the image whilst air, being least dense, appears black. Since electron density is the only measurement parameter, radiographic and CT appearances are consistent, predictable and, therefore, reproducible. In MRI, however, there are a number of measurement parameters which affect signal intensity and, subsequently, image contrast. This means that the operator can manipulate image contrast to the extent of turning the appearance of water, for example, from black to white. This may appear confusing until the principles are understood. In fact, it is the ability to manipulate contrast in this way that gives MRI its superior soft tissue differentiation.

Later, consideration will be given to how the operator can alter scan parameters in order to produce these changes in image contrast but first of all we should explore the hydrogen proton, how MRI uses radiofrequency (RF) energy to produce resonance and what happens as the proton relaxes when the RF pulse is turned off.

The hydrogen proton

There are several atoms that possess the ability to resonate and can be used to produce images. In fact any atom with an odd mass number such as carbon (13), sodium (23) and phosphorous (31) would be suitable, but in clinical use only hydrogen, with a mass number of one, is used. This is because a single hydrogen atom produces a relatively large magnetic moment and resonates very well; it is said to have a high **gyromagnetic ratio** (γ) and it is abundant within the body.

Hydrogen is the simplest of atoms, having a nucleus composed of a single proton (no neutrons) and has no orbiting electrons; hence it is often referred to simply as a proton.

The proton carries a positive electrical charge and spins on its own axis. This moving electrical charge, according to the laws of electromagnetic induction, creates a corresponding magnetic field around the proton so that it behaves like a tiny bar magnet having north and south poles (Figure 1.1). Such magnetic fields are described in physics as magnetic moments. Each magnetic

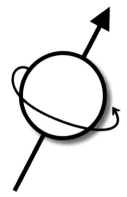

Figure 1.1 The hydrogen proton.

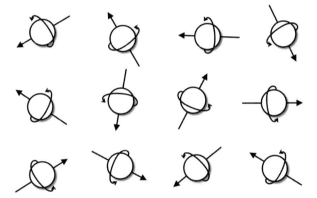

Figure 1.2 In the normal state of affairs magnetic moments are randomly orientated and cancel each other out.

moment possesses the properties of size and direction. Where two or more magnetic moments exist together, their size and direction (or vectors) can be combined to give their net magnetisation. Thus if two magnetic moments exist both having the same size and direction their net magnetisation will be double that of each individual. Conversely if they have the same size but opposite direction the two will cancel each other out and their net magnetisation will be zero. In the normal course of events the body's many billions of microscopic magnetic moments are completely randomly orientated (Figure 1.2) and cancel each other out such that their macroscopic or net magnetic field is zero.

The effects of an external magnetic field B_0

When an animal is placed into the MRI scanner, the external magnetic field (referred to as B_0) causes the protons to abandon their random orientation and 'line up' with the main magnetic field. Current knowledge of magnets and magnetic fields would suggest that the tiny magnetic fields of each proton would adopt an orientation parallel to the main field B_0 with their north and south poles matching those of the main magnet. However the laws of quantum mechanics dictate that certain protons have sufficient thermal energy at room temperature to adopt an opposing, anti-parallel state. Indeed the two populations are almost identical. Moreover the protons are continually oscillating between the two states but at any given point in time, the ratio of anti-parallel to parallel states is one million to one million and six at a B_0 field strength of 1 Tesla (1 T). This excess population of six in one million means that our patient's total hydrogen content has a **net magnetisation vector** (NMV) in the parallel direction (Figure 1.3). With only six in two million protons contributing to the image it seems doubtful that the process will work at all. However, at 1.5 T 0.01 ml of water contains around 3 million billion such excess protons, so things begin to seem feasible.

Since the energy level required to achieve the anti-parallel state increases with the field strength of B_0, and the patient's thermal energy remains fairly constant, it follows that the magnitude of the NMV increases with the field strength of the MRI system we

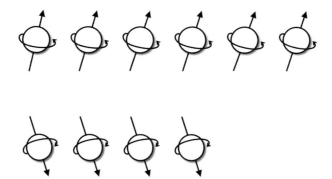

Figure 1.3 The influence of an external magnetic field is to align protons in the parallel and anti-parallel states.

are using. This is an important relationship, since it is the NMV that contributes the useful MRI signal. Hence systems with high field strength magnets generate more signal from the same volume of tissue than lower field systems.

A second influence of B_0 is to cause spinning protons to **precess**. Just as a child's spinning top begins to wobble under the influence of gravity, so protons are made to wobble or precess by B_0. The exact frequency of this precession is given by the Larmor equation:

$$\omega_0 = B_0\gamma$$

where ω_0 can be referred to as the Larmor, precessional or resonant frequency and γ is the gyromagnetic ratio referred to earlier in this chapter and is a constant unique to each atom. Since γ is constant for hydrogen, it can be seen from this equation that precessional frequency is directly linked to field strength B_0 thus:

- The precessional frequency of hydrogen at 1.0 T is 42.57 MHz.
- Therefore its precessional frequency at 0.5 T will be 21.285 MHz.

The exact equation does not have to be remembered, but this is an important relationship to grasp as it will help the understanding of a number of other concepts which follow.

The major effect of this precessional motion is to introduce a transverse component to the magnetic field of each proton since each is now spinning at a slight tilt to B_0 (Figure 1.4). Because the north/south poles of each proton are pointing in random directions at any one time (Figure 1.5), they still cancel each other out in the transverse plane so that the NMV is still in the parallel or longitudinal direction.

The effects of an RF pulse at the Larmor frequency: resonance

If a pulse of radiofrequency (RF) energy is now applied to protons in the system it can cause the hydrogen spins to react to it provided two important conditions are fulfilled. These are that the RF pulse must be applied at right angles to B_0 and that it must be

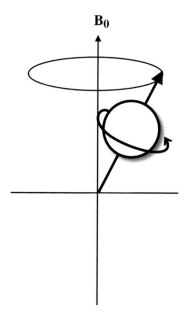

Figure 1.4 Precession.

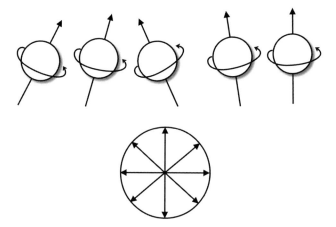

Figure 1.5 Out of phase in the transverse plane.

at the Larmor frequency; any other frequency at this field strength will have no effect on hydrogen.

This reaction to the RF pulse is **resonance** and, essentially, two things happen. One is that the RF pulse imparts sufficient energy to allow more protons to adopt the anti-parallel state The six

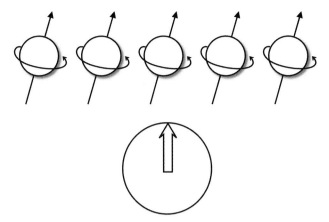

Figure 1.6 In phase in the transverse plane.

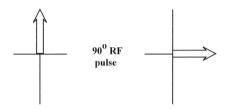

Figure 1.7 Net magnetisation passes through 90° from longitudinal to transverse planes.

excess protons discussed earlier provide an illustration of what happens if enough RF energy is transmitted to allow three of these to flip into the anti- parallel position. They will then cancel out the other three in the parallel state and the NMV in the longitudinal plane will now be zero. The other effect, which takes place in the transverse plane, is to bring all our hydrogen spins into phase with each other. Now, instead of all the spins cancelling each other out, each microscopic magnetic field is in unison with its neighbours; they are said to be 'in phase' (Figure 1.6).

Consequently their individual magnetic fields all add together so that the NMV is now at a maximum in the transverse plane. The NMV has shifted through 90° from longitudinal to transverse. If the RF transmission is terminated at this point it is said to be a **90° RF pulse** (Figure 1.7). Note that the angle through which the NMV tilts or the 'flip angle' (α), in this case 90°, is a function of the strength and duration of the RF pulse. Other values for α will be encountered later.

And when the RF transmission is turned off …

Three things begin to happen simultaneously but independently of each other as soon as the RF transmission is turned off. Each will be considered in some detail but briefly what happens is this:

1. Because the NMV is now in the transverse plane and no longer overwhelmed by B_0 it can be detected by a receiver coil. The absorbed RF energy is retransmitted as the useable MR signal. How much signal is transmitted will depend on how much hydrogen there is in a particular tissue; its **proton density** (PD).
2. The spins that were in phase with each other in the transverse plane are affected to varying degrees by other atoms locally and some begin to slow down relative to others; they begin to **dephase**. This is referred to as **T2 relaxation**, also called transverse or spin spin relaxation.
3. The extra protons that were able to use RF energy to adopt the anti-parallel state are now reliant again on thermal energy alone and begin to return to their usual state, thermal equilibrium. This, surprisingly enough, is called **T1 relaxation**. This process is also referred to as longitudinal recovery or spin lattice relaxation.

Transmission of the MR signal

The concept of electromagnetic induction teaches that a moving magnetic field will induce an electrical current in an adjacent conductor. That is exactly the situation in the spin system; the rotating magnetic field in the transverse plane will produce an electromagnetic radiation at the Larmor frequency. It is this RF emission that gives the useable MR signal that goes to make up the final image. The amount of signal generated by various tissues within the body is determined by the amount of hydrogen each contains, as well as their T1 and T2 relaxation times. Tissues containing lots of hydrogen such as fat and cerebrospinal fluid (CSF) will generate lots of signal. Conversely tissues like cortical bone and lung, which contain little or no hydrogen, will generate very low signal or even a signal void.

By placing a suitable receiver coil (discussed later) close to the patient the signals being emitted can be collected for conversion into shades of grey in the MR image.

T1 relaxation (longitudinal recovery)

Once the RF pulse is turned off, it no longer contributes energy to the spin system. In the absence of any external influence the hydrogen spins will return to their thermal equilibrium. Their acquired energy is given off partly as emitted RF radiation but mostly as heat to the surrounding tissues, or **lattice**. Hence T1 relaxation is sometimes referred to as spin lattice relaxation. This results in an exponential regrowth in longitudinal magnetisation (Figure 1.8). T1 relaxation time itself is defined as the time taken for 63% of magnetisation to realign with B_0. This relaxation

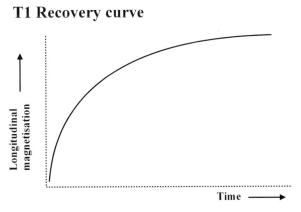

T1 Recovery curve

Longitudinal magnetisation

Time

Figure 1.8 Recovery of longitudinal magnetisation.

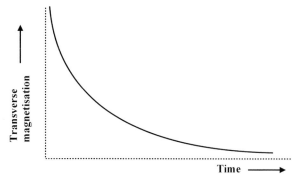

T2 Decay curve

Figure 1.9 Decay of transverse magnetisation.

process is called recovery since it represents a return to maximum from zero.

T2 relaxation (transverse decay)

At the point that the RF pulse is terminated, all spins in the transverse plan are spinning in-phase with each other; in the absence of this overriding influence, protons begin to be influenced by the magnetic fields of neighbouring atoms. This will make some protons to begin to spin more slowly than their neighbours causing them to get out of synchronisation with each other; in other words the spin system begins to **dephase**. This causes signals in the transverse plane to start to cancel each other out leading to an exponential loss of signal from transverse magnetisation (Figure 1.9). Again note that T2 relaxation is called decay since it represents a loss of signal from maximum to zero.

Free induction decay

The term free induction decay, or FID for short, is used to describe what happens to the current induced in the receiver coil at the end of the RF pulse provided no other influences are brought to bear. In the perfect world this would follow the T2 decay curve but, in reality, FID is also affected by inhomogeneities in the MR

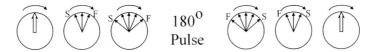

Figure 1.10 180° RF pulse serves to refocus dephasing protons (F = fast, S = slow).

system and so is said to portray the T2* (pronounced T2 star) decay function. These inhomogeneities arise from many sources, for example imperfections in manufacture; metal within the patient (surgical clips, id chips etc.); gradient fields applied as part of the MR process, to name but a few.

The good news is that these field inhomogeneities can be compensated for to give us a true T2 relaxation curve. This is done by applying a second RF pulse, having twice the energy of the first, at some point after dephasing has occurred. This is described as a 180° RF pulse as it has the effect of flipping the NMV through 180°. This reversal of the spin system has the effect of swapping fast and slow precessing protons (Figure 1.10) such that faster protons now begin to catch up with slower ones so that they come back into phase rebuilding signal to produce an **echo** (this is discussed further in the next section). Since true T2 decay also affects the rephasing process, the echo has a lower magnitude than the original FID. This reduction in magnitude reflects the true T2 relaxation curve. The time (TE) at which the echo is produced can be predetermined by altering the time ($^{TE}/_2$) at which the 180° pulse is applied. When spatial encoding of signals is considered it will explain why this process of echo formation needs to be repeated many times to give enough information to produce an image. For now let's look at how the repetition time (TR) and echo time (TE) can be altered to manipulate contrast in the final image.

Image weighting and contrast

Spin echo sequences

In the last section it was seen that dephasing in the transverse plane was not simply a function of true T2 relaxation but was also affected by inhomogeneities in the MR system; the, so called, T2* effect. It would obviously be advantageous if these two processes could be separated to give a true T2 representation in our final image. This can be achieved as described above by using an additional RF pulse which, this time, produces a 180° shift of the NMV. The affect of this 180° RF pulse is best appreciated by considering it in two 90° portions. The first 90° will bring spins back into phase (just as the original 90° pulse did) whilst the second will continue to push spins out of phase but in the opposite direction so that, although still precessing in the same direction, fast moving spins now find themselves behind slow moving ones, with the result that, once the RF pulse has been turned off, they gradually catch up. The spins are said to rephrase or refocus (Figure 1.10). A corresponding regrowth of signal is detected in the receiver coil, referred to as an echo. Inhomogeneities remain unchanged so their effects are 'ironed out' but since true T2 influences are still at work during the refocusing period, the echo doesn't have quite the same amplitude as the FID so the echo is a representation of the true T2 relaxation function (Figure 1.11).

This refocusing process forms the basis of spin echo (SE) pulse sequences and manipulation of the timing of these 90° and 180° RF pulses determines image contrast.

A single echo is not sufficient to give an image. In practice, for purposes of spatial localisation, the whole process is repeated hundreds of times. The time between one 90° RF pulse and the

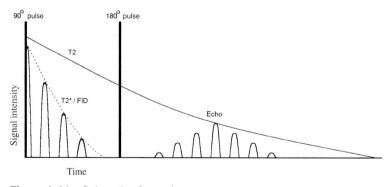

Figure 1.11 Spin echo formation.

T2 relaxation

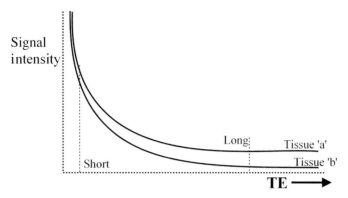

Figure 1.12 T2 contrast is more obvious at longer TE times.

next is referred to as the **repetition time** or TR whilst the time taken for an echo to form is called the echo time or TE. By altering TR and TE we can manipulate image contrast.

First let's examine the effects of altering the echo time, TE. Consider the T2 decay curve from earlier in this chapter. In Figure 1.12 the T2 curves for two different tissues (a and b) are shown. If an echo is produced with a relatively short TE (echo time is determined by the time at which the 180° RF pulse is applied) then it can be seen from the diagram that there is little contrast between the two tissues. Compare this to the much better degree of contrast evident using a longer TE. In summary we can say that the length of TE affects contrast as follows:

- A long TE: maximises T2 contrast.
- A short TE: minimises T2 contrast.

Now a comparison may be made of the T1 recovery curves for the same two tissues (Figure 1.13) together with an examination of the effects of using a long and short TR. If we choose to wait a long time before repeating the 90° pulse then both tissues will have had time to relax completely so that when the next 90° RF pulse is applied it will produce maximum transverse magnetisation

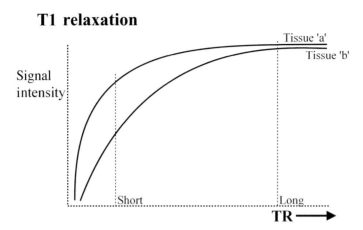

Figure 1.13 T1 contrast is more obvious at shorter TR times.

in both tissues, thereby giving little or no contrast between them. Choosing a shorter TR on the other hand means that tissue b has only partially recovered so that, when the 90° RF pulse is repeated on this occasion, tissue a will give maximum transverse magnetisation while tissue b will only produce a portion of this, resulting in a contrast between the two tissues. Again to summarise:

- A long TR: minimises T1 contrast.
- A short TR: maximises T1 contrast.

The two relaxation processes, T1 and T2, although occurring simultaneously, are completely independent of each other and so the two can never be separated. By choosing the correct combination of TE and TR as outlined above, however, the sequence can be optimised in favour of the desired contrast. The resultant images are said to be either T1 or T2 **weighted** and commonly expressed as T1W or T2W.

Using the observations so far, the following combinations can be put together:

- A short TR maximises T1 contrast while a short TE minimises T2.
- Short TR and short TE give T1 weighting (T1W).

- A long TR minimises T1 contrast while a long TE maximises T2.
- Long TR and long TE give T2 weighting (T2W).

A third combination can be used to minimise both T1 and T2 effects. At first this may seem to be rather a counter-productive thing to want to do but remember that tissues with differing amounts of hydrogen in their composition will produce different amounts of signal. Any contrast in this image is down to absolute numbers of hydrogen atoms rather than either of the relaxation processes. Such an image is said to be **proton density weighted** (PDW).

- A long TR minimises T1 contrast and a short TE minimises T2.
- Long TR and short TE give proton density weighting (PDW).

There is, of course, a fourth combination available, that of short TR and long TE. The discussions thus far would suggest that such a combination would attempt to optimise both T1 and T2 at the same time. Experimenting with such a combination will clearly show that this is not a desirable combination, resulting in images of very poor quality that show no useful information.

Table 1.1 summarises the options for tissue contrast weighting in spin echo imaging and gives some typical TR and TE values in milliseconds (ms).

Table 1.1 Options for tissue contrast weighting in spin echo imaging, with some typical TR and TE values in milliseconds (ms).

	TR	TE	Fat	Water
T1W	Short 300–600 ms	Short 10–20 ms	High signal (bright)	Low signal (dark)
T2W	Long >2000 ms	Long 90–120 ms	High signal (bright)	High signal (bright)
PDW	Long >2000 ms	Short 15–25 ms	High signal (bright)	High signal (bright)*

*Water should appear bright on PDW images since it contains lots of hydrogen but requires very long TR values to allow full T1 relaxation. At values around 2000 ms water may still appear dark.

BASIC PRINCIPLES

Pulse sequences

Contrast mechanisms also vary according to the type of pulse sequence that is used. A pulse sequence, as the name would suggest, describes the sequence and timing of RF pulses and gradient applications required to produce an image. So far, to illustrate the basic T1, T2 and PD contrast mechanisms, the straightforward SE sequence has been used. As described earlier, this uses a 90° RF pulse followed by a 180° RF pulse to produce an echo. There are, however, other combinations or sequences which can be used either to produce alternative contrast characteristics or to speed up the process of image production. These will be examined in more detail in the rest of this chapter, but the basic principles of SE image contrast are perhaps most valuable in understanding contrast mechanisms.

The number and exact mechanism of pulse sequences available, particularly on sophisticated modern systems, are many. Each manufacturer is continually developing new pulse sequences in an attempt to keep abreast of the competition in terms of speed and image quality. To try to describe each and every pulse sequence available is beyond the scope of this book but a few sequences are worth mentioning in general terms either because of their unique contrast or the increase in speed of image acquisition they afford.

Inversion recovery

One such sequence worthy of some consideration at this stage is **inversion recovery** (IR) as it provides some unique types of contrast encountered in every day use. IR differs from SE in that it starts with a 180° RF inversion pulse (Figure 1.14) then allows a period of relaxation or recovery; this period being known as the inversion time (TI). The TI is then followed by a standard SE sequence as described above. Originally used to produce heavily T1 weighted images, inversion recovery is more often encountered nowadays as either STIR (short time inversion recovery) or FLAIR (fluid attenuated inversion recovery) sequences. By manipulating the TI period (Figure 1.15), the SE part of the sequence can be started at a point where the longitudinal recovery curve passes through zero, the so-called null point. This means that no magne-

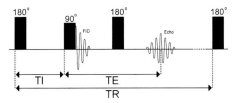

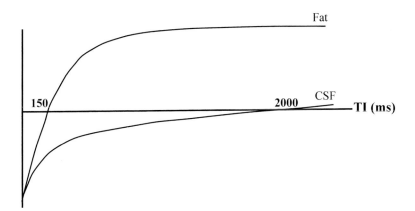

Figure 1.14 Inversion recovery sequence.

Figure 1.15 Basis of the STIR sequence.

tisation will be flipped into the transverse plane by the 90° pulse and, consequently, no signal will be returned by the receiver coil. Since different tissues have different T1 recovery times, we can choose a TI to match the null point of a particular tissue.

In STIR imaging a short TI is used (around 160 ms at 1.0 T) which corresponds to the null point of fat. The resultant images show no signal from fat, which would normally be bright on conventional SE sequences. This is particularly useful when trying to demonstrate lesions in parts of the body such as the abdomen or orbits which contain lots of fat. Eliminating signal from fat will inevitably lead to a reduction in signal to noise ratio (SNR) (more of this later) producing rather 'noisy' images but, since most pathology tends to be high in water content, lesions on STIR images tend to stand out against the darker fat-free background (Figure 1.16).

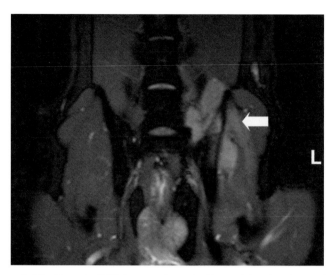

Figure 1.16 Dorsal STIR image through the pelvis showing a lesion adjacent to the iliac wing (arrow). Note that normal fatty marrow is rendered low signal intensity, emphasising invasion of the ilium on the left side.

FLAIR uses a much longer TI (2000 ms) which coincides with the null point of water so that FLAIR images show low signal intensity in areas of free fluid. Bound fluid, on the other hand, has a quicker relaxation time because it is able to impart energy to the molecules to which it is bound. Consequently areas of oedema, tumour, necrosis or other pathology will retain a high signal, whilst areas of free fluid, such as CSF, will appear dark. This is a particularly useful sequence in imaging of the brain where it demonstrates periventricular lesions which may otherwise have been obscured by high signal from CSF.

Spin echo and scan time

It should now be apparent that SE sequences, including inversion recovery, involve repeated applications of the 90° and 180° RF pulses, commonly as many as 512 times or more. Given that a

T2W scan sequence requires a TR of at least 2000 ms (2 s), then the scan time for this sequence would be (512 × 2) seconds or 17 minutes! In short, conventional SE sequences (especially for T2W) are very slow. Clearly there was a need to develop sequences that could give adequate contrast weighting but greatly improve scan speed.

Before looking at how the problems of scan speed have been addressed, it would be helpful to understand just why so many repetitions are required. The answer lies in how the MR signal is spatially localised.

Spatial localisation

So far in this chapter it has been shown how the MR signal is produced and how, by manipulating TR and TE, the image contrast can be influenced. In order to convert these signals into a meaningful image, however, we also need to know from where in the patient they originate. In other words they need to be spatially localised. Once this is known the various signal intensities can be converted to shades of grey to fill in the picture elements, or pixels, and the picture then is complete. As in other kinds of digital imaging the pixels are the 'dots' which make up the image. In MRI, however, the image represents a slice of tissue within the patient so the shade of grey allocated to a pixel represents the signal intensities of a three-dimensional picture element called a **voxel** (Figure 1.17).

The first requirement is to be able to select an imaging slice in terms of its orthogonal plane and its thickness.

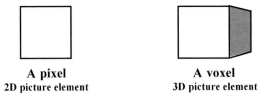

A pixel
2D picture element

A voxel
3D picture element

Figure 1.17 Area resolution is represented by pixels, spatial resolution by voxels.

Slice location

It should be remembered from the Larmor equation that resonance only takes place at the Larmor frequency and this is dependent on magnetic field strength. If, instead of a uniform magnetic
field, the scanner's magnetic field strength were to vary from one
end to the other, then this would be referred to as applying a
magnetic field **gradient** (Figure 1.18a). In this example, if an RF

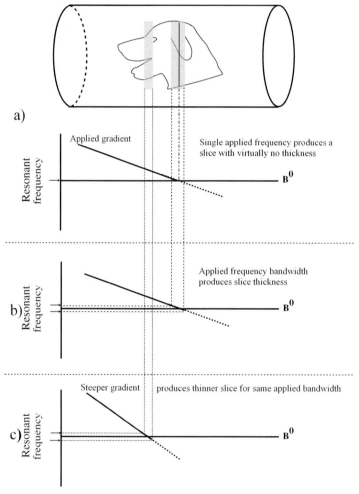

Figure 1.18 Using applied gradients to select slice location and
thickness.

pulse is applied at the resonant frequency for B_0, protons will only resonate at the point along the gradient where it is equal to B_0. At any other point the field strength will be higher or lower than B_0 and so resonance will not occur.

If a single RF frequency is used the resultant slice which is excited will have virtually no thickness. In order to give the slice thickness, it is necessary to excite a range of frequencies (Figure 1.18b). This range is referred to as the excitation **bandwidth**. The slice thickness can be altered by changing the bandwidth or the steepness of the gradient as shown in Figure 1.18c.

In this example a transverse section has been selected by applying the gradient along the z axis. Sagittal and dorsal orientations can be obtained by using the x and y gradients (Figure 1.19), whilst oblique sections employ a combination of axes. Once slice selection has been performed, some way of determining where within the slice the various signal intensities should be plotted in the image is still needed. They require the equivalent of a map reference.

Frequency encoding

In order to convert the various signal intensities emanating from the selected slice of the patient into a sensible image, it is essential to be able to convert their position in the patient into a cor-

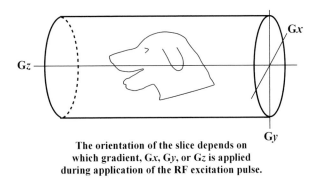

The orientation of the slice depends on
which gradient, Gx, Gy, or Gz is applied
during application of the RF excitation pulse.

Figure 1.19 Slice orientation depends on the combination of applied gradients.

responding position on the image. The analogy of the map reference here is a good one. If each image element (pixel) is given such a 'map reference' (equivalent to longitude and latitude) it can be given a position on the image grid or **matrix**.

In the previous section on slice location we have seen that protons can be easily located by giving them specific frequency encoding. In the example used to demonstrate slice location a gradient was applied along the z axis. This leaves two other axes, x and y, to be encoded. This can be done along one axis by applying another gradient just before the echo signal is collected. If a gradient is applied along the x axis just before the echo is collected in the receiver coil, instead of all the protons precessing at the same frequency, they will now have different frequencies dependent on their position along the x axis gradient. Using this gradient technique the x direction of the image matrix can be divided into frequency encoded columns but it is still necessary to encode the signal in the other matrix direction. Using a second gradient in the y axis would seem the simple solution but this would result in protons from different parts of the image having the same frequency.

Phase encoding

The solution is to apply a gradient very briefly after the slice has been excited but before the frequency encoding gradient is applied. This has the effect of changing the frequency of precession but only for a split second before returning it to the original state. This brief 'blip' has the effect of changing the angle of precession or phase. If a different steepness of gradient (using negative as well as positive values) is applied for each repetition then the signal collected at any one point during each TR will be different. Although each will have the same frequency (because the position along the frequency encoding gradient has not changed) the signal for each TR will be slightly out of phase with every other TR. In effect a number of phase-encoded rows have been produced. Note however, that each phase encoding step requires an additional TR so the more phase encoding steps acquired the longer the final scan time will be. This relationship between image matrix and scan time will be discussed in more detail in Chapter 3 but at this point it is worth noting that the more encoding steps there are in both the frequency and phase directions, the more pixels there will be in the final image and hence resolution will improve.

Fourier transformation

Now that signal strength can be measured and the position of signals plotted on a matrix, all that remains is to convert these digital signal values into shades of grey and an image is produced. This conversion is achieved using a complex mathematical process called **2D Fourier transform**. Fourier transform takes the digital data held in 'K space' (a mathematical model used to represent the information held in the computer's memory and little to do with real space) and converts it into an accurate geometrical representation of tissues within the imaging slice.

Pulse sequences: the quest for speed

The relationship between the number of phase encoding steps, scan time and image resolution should now be becoming clearer. More phase encoding steps mean more pixels and better resolution but at the expense of longer scan times. Two major advances in pulse sequence technology were to bring about vastly improved performance in terms of scan times. The first of these was **gradient echo** (GE), followed some years later by **fast spin echo** (FSE).

Gradient echo

Although today's gradient echo pulse sequences are many and varied and often very complex, the basic principle was very straightforward. Instead of allowing nature to take its course and waiting for protons to dephase then applying a 180° RF pulse and waiting for them to rephase generating an echo, gradient echo intervened

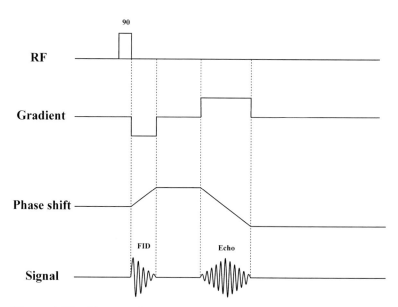

Figure 1.20 Diagramatic representation of the gradient echo pulse sequence.

to speed up the whole process. The description of spatial encoding has shown that the application of a field gradient will make protons precess at different speeds. This variation in precessional speed will, in turn, lead to dephasing of protons. The gradient echo sequence in its most basic form simply applies a gradient to forcibly dephase spins then reverses the gradient to produce an echo (Figure 1.20). The result is a dramatic reduction in scan time. In the absence of the 180° RF refocusing pulse found in SE sequences, however, there is no longer any compensation for field inhomogeneities. In fact field inhomogeneities (in the form of gradients) are deliberately used as part of the pulse sequence. As a result, gradient echo sequences are said to produce T2* (pronounced T2 star) weighted images rather than true T2W.

Fast spin echo

The development of FSE sequences was a major breakthrough in MR imaging. Also referred to by some manufacturers as turbo spin

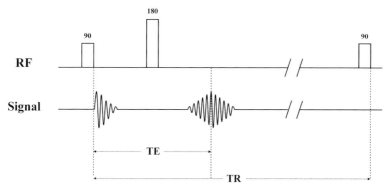

Figure 1.21 Diagramatic representation of the spin echo pulse sequence.

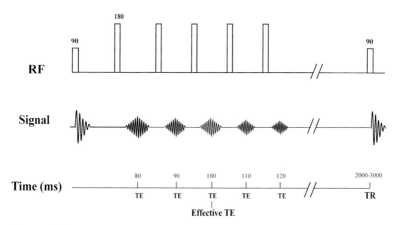

Figure 1.22 Diagramatic representation of the turbo spin echo pulse sequence.

echo (TSE), fast spin echo (FSE) offered a considerable reduction in scan times whilst producing image contrast that was very close to true T2W.

In conventional SE sequences (Figure 1.21), one phase encoding is produced during each TR period. FSE achieves faster scan times by acquiring multiple phase encoding steps per TR. Figure 1.22 shows five phase encodings being acquired in a single TR period. In this example, scan speed will increase by a factor of five since five phase encoding steps are being carried out for every one in a conventional SE sequence. This number is referred to as the echo train length (ETL); also referred to by some manufacturers as the turbo factor. In practice an ETL of 20 or more is commonly used for T2W FSE sequences giving a massive boost in terms of scanning speed. For this reason virtually all T2W sequences encountered in current routine clinical practice will be FSE.

2 MR System Hardware

As seen in the previous chapter, there are several steps involved in getting from a spinning proton to a meaningful MR image, requiring a whole range of elaborate hardware along the way. This chapter will consider the main components of the MR system, what they do and how they influence the end product. As well as helping to understand the whole process, this chapter should help in making a choice of a system or service appropriate to individual circumstances.

Magnets

Probably the most obvious component is a magnet since this is at the heart of any MR system, large or small. There are many types of magnet with a great variety of applications, e.g. navigational compasses, fridge door magnets, etc.

Magnetic field strength is measured in units called Gauss (G) and Tesla (T): 10 000 G = 1 T. To put these measurements into some sort of perspective, the earth's magnetic field is about 5 G, depending where on the earth's surface it is measured. A scrapyard car-lifting magnet, on the other hand, measures around 1 T.

In MRI systems the main types on offer are permanent, resistive and superconducting magnets. In veterinary practice it is most likely that either a permanent or a superconducting magnet will be installed in the system. The resistive type is essentially an electromagnet like the scrapyard variety. It has the advantage that it can be easily turned off when not in use but it has fallen from favour because of its need for electricity to maintain the field. This makes such systems expensive to run.

Permanent magnets

Permanent magnets, as the name would suggest, are made of a permanently magnetic material such as iron or ceramic. The field strength of these systems is severely limited by the sheer weight of the core. Consequently, permanent magnet systems operate at low field strength, typically around 0.25 T (Figure 2.1). Using a

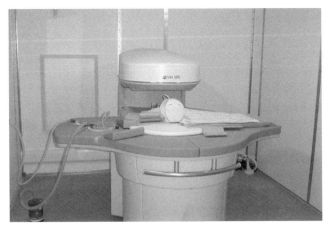

Figure 2.1 Low field (0.18 T) MRI system – Esaote.

permanent magnet makes low field systems relatively inexpensive to buy and cheap to run, also their small fringe field makes them safer than high field systems. In Chapter 1 MR signal was seen to increase with field strength. The low field strength of permanent MR scanners brings with it limitations in terms of image quality, whilst the smaller size can place restrictions on the size of animal that can be accommodated. They are, however, perfectly adequate and produce good results when scanning dogs and cats. Their size, cost and servicing requirements add to their attractiveness for large referral practices with competent staff.

Superconducting magnets

Strictly speaking these are electromagnets but of a rather special kind. Their magnetic field is produced by passing a current through conducting wire loops made of a titanium alloy. These windings are immersed in an insulated jacket of liquid helium at a temperature of almost absolute zero (liquid helium boils at 4 K). At temperatures below 9.5 K the titanium alloy windings have no resistance to current flow. Consequently, once the field has been built up gradually to the required level, the power supply can be turned off and the current will continue to flow *ad infinitum*. Despite being a resistive magnet, by removing the resistance in this way, the superconducting magnet also becomes permanent. It is essential to remember that any type of magnet encountered in veterinary MRI is likely to have its field *always on*, even when not in use and the rest of the system is turned off.

Because there is no heavy core involved, superconducting magnets can achieve very high field strengths: 1–1.5 T (Figure 2.2) is usual for both human and veterinary use and in the human field research machines of up to 7.0 T are capable of whole body imaging.

Needless to say, machines of this size are much more expensive to buy and their requirement for a special power supply can add to initial installation costs even for visits by a mobile unit. Maintenance costs, including the need to top up the liquid helium regularly, are high and, as with any complex equipment, breakdowns are not uncommon.

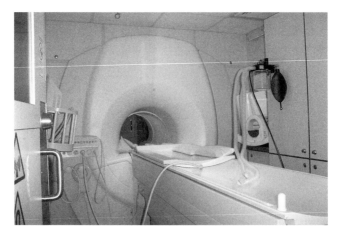

Figure 2.2 High field (1.0 T) MRI system – Philips Medical Systems.

Shielding

At these high field strengths it is crucial to limit the external or **fringe** field as this contributes nothing to image formation and is potentially hazardous since fields in excess of 5 G can cause cardiac pacemakers to malfunction. If the fringe field greater than 5 G can be contained within the scan room itself, then pacemaker wearers can easily be excluded. Fringe fields can also interfere with anything that uses magnetism, such as credit cards, computer screens and other sensitive equipment. It should be noted however that the magnet's ability to attract ferromagnetic objects (the 'missile' effect) is not overcome by sheilding. Potential missiles will not be attracted from such distances as they may have been by the fringe field but they will be attacted by the main field with greater acceleration since the distance between 5 G and 1.5 T (for example) is now shorter. In other words the gradient is steeper.

Passive shielding involves placing a physical iron shield around the magnet to limit the fringe field. This is a simple, fairly effective method but adds considerably to the weight of the scanner. Another very effective way of substantially reducing fringe fields is to use active shielding. This involves adding a second set of superconducting coils outside the primary one but wound in the opposite direction.

Shimming

For the MR process to work at all requires an absolutely uniform (homogeneous) magnetic field. To achieve this, a series of up to 30 additional wire coils sited just inside the main magnet bore are used. Passing currents through these additional **shim coils** allows the field to be 'tweaked' to make it as homogeneous as possible. Further **active shimming** can also be carried out (usually automatically) prior to each examination to compensate for inhomogeneities introduced by the patient.

Gradients

The last chapter demonstrated the important role gradients play in encoding the image and controlling the various steps of each pulse sequence. Three sets of gradient coils (in practice a pair of gradient coils is needed to produce a linear magnetic field gradient) *x, y* and *z* are employed. These three gradient orientations correspond in imaging terms to the three orthogonal planes: sagittal, transverse and dorsal of the patient.

The specification of gradient coils can have a significant effect on the overall performance of any MR system. Essentially there are two important properties to consider. The **peak amplitude**, measured in milliTesla per metre (mT/m), indicates the maximum steepness of gradient achievable. Steep gradients (25–30 mT/m) are important, particularly when scanning small animals, in achieving thin slices, small field of view etc. Equally important is the time taken for gradient coils to reach their peak amplitude. This is the, so called, **rise time** or **slew rate** and is expressed in mT/m/ms. High rise times are essential for fast imaging techniques but this is less of a concern in veterinary imaging where the patients are anaesthetised. It could, however, be a consideration in abdominal examinations where there is a need to reduce physiological motion artefact.

Radiofrequency system

The excitation radiofrequency (RF) pulse is transmitted (with only one or two exceptions) by the body coil which is housed, along with the gradient coils, inside the scanner itself. Consequently the operator has no direct influence over the transmitted RF pulse. The same is not true, however, about the receiver coils used to detect signal coming from the patient: the echo.

The choice of receiver coil can have a dramatic effect on SNR. At first this may appear a little odd since the amount of signal available is determined by the patient: volume of tissue, proton density and tissue relaxation constants T1 and T2. It follows, therefore, that the choice of coil cannot influence the amount of signal detected. Figure 2.3, however, shows that the choice of coil can dramatically reduce the amount of noise collected, thereby increasing SNR. Generally speaking, the receiver coil chosen should be the smallest available, consistent with including the anatomy to be examined. It is also worth noting that when using surface coils, i.e. coils which do not completely surround the

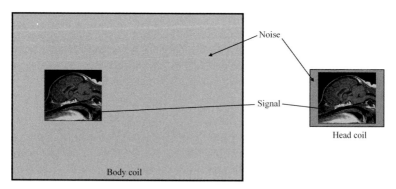

Figure 2.3 How reciever coil selection affects signal to noise ratio (SNR). Both coils collect the same amount of signal but the head coil collects less noise, making its SNR much better.

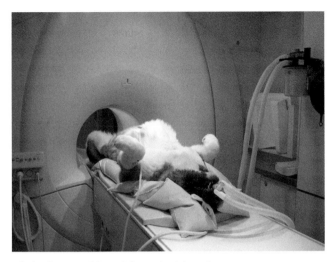

Figure 2.4 Dog positioned for spinal imaging.

patient, signal intensity falls away with distance from the coil so that it is important to have the region being examined close to the coil. Using a spinal phased array coil, for example, animals are best scanned in dorsal recumbency so that the spinal column is as close to the receiver coil as possible (Figure 2.4).

Faraday cage

The MRI process is heavily dependant on the use of RF. The RF used is at frequencies in line with those employed in everyday use for various radio transmissions. Consequently the scanner must be housed in a room which protects it from external RF transmissions. This is achieved by shielding the room using a 'Faraday cage' which, provided the door is firmly closed, will prevent RF waves from entering the scanning room and being detected by the receiver coils, thereby creating artefact (see Chapter 4). The Faraday cage is an earthed enclosure constructed from fine metallic mesh or foil which encompasses the entire scan room including the door and window(s) thus intercepting and earthing incoming radio waves.

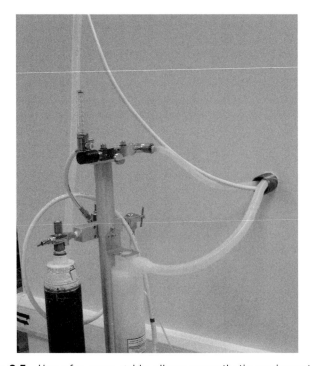

Figure 2.5 Use of a wave guide allows anaesthetic equipment to be positioned outside the scan room.

Access to the room for anaesthetic tubing and monitoring cables is provided via a special port called a 'wave guide' (Figure 2.5). This allows tubing and cables to be passed through the scan room wall without allowing radio waves to pass, thus maintaining the integrity of the Faraday cage.

Image processing and archiving

The final link in the hardware chain is the computing and archiving elements. As with most computing tasks, big is best. At the end of each scan sequence, a large amount of data is presented for reconstruction into recognisable images. If the system's computer is lacking in processing power irritating delays can occur whilst images are reconstructed ready for viewing. Finally, once images have been created, some form of long-term storage or archiving is required. Many systems use magneto-optical discs (MODs) but it is becoming increasingly common for newer systems to use CDs or even DVDs as a cheap and easy means of storing images.

MR SYSTEM HARDWARE

3 Imaging Parameters

The objective when carrying out MRI, or any other imaging procedure for that matter, should be to produce good-quality images in
a reasonable examination time. This chapter will explore what
constitutes a good image and how the various scan measurement
parameters can be manipulated to achieve this objective. In addition, consideration will be given to the impact various parameters
have on each other and on image acquisition time.

Three main elements come together to form a 'good' image,
they are **signal**, **resolution** and **contrast**. Image quality can also
be degraded by the presence of **artefacts**. Unfortunately, when
selecting imaging parameters, we can never optimise all of these
constituent parts at the same time. Invariably, improving one
component will lead to degradation of another – the so-called
'trade-off'. Furthermore, it is apparent from Chapter 1 that many
of the parameters available have an impact on scan time. It is up
to the competent practitioner to decide which element(s) are
important for a particular sequence or examination and select
parameters accordingly to optimise a particular element or elements of image quality in an acceptable timeframe. For example,
in abdominal imaging minimising artefacts from physiological
motion is important, whereas examination of the pituitary requires
high resolution.

Signal and noise

- Signal – arises from protons that were excited intentionally.
- Noise – comes from hydrogen protons and other MR active nuclei that are moving from high to low energy levels due to random thermal activity along with random signal generated by the MR system.

Clearly, signal is a desirable quality in the final image whilst noise is not. The objectives when selecting scan parameters, therefore, should be to maximise signal and/or to minimise noise. Best images are produced when the level of signal is high relative to the level of noise. This relationship is quantified as the signal to noise ratio or SNR and is calculated by dividing average signal by the standard deviation of noise.

The amount of signal produced is dependent on **tissue parameters**, **measurement parameters** and **system parameters**. Tissue parameters (proton density, T1 and T2 relaxation constants) are patient dependent and the operator has no control over these, but it should be remembered that larger animals produce more signal than smaller ones (they contain more protons). Likewise, since fat is high signal on T1W, T2W and PDW images, fatter animals will give more signal than lean or undernourished ones. Experience has also shown that some patients, for whatever reason, appear to resonate better than others.

Measurement parameters

These are the factors over which the operator has control. They are:

- pulse parameters – TR, TE, TI, flip angle;
- slice parameters – slice thickness and slice gap;
- matrix size;
- signal averages;
- bandwidth (or more accurately, receive bandwidth).

Each of these factors affects the signal generated by the MR system.

Repetition time

From the Chapter 1 it will be remembered that if a TR is long enough it will allow complete longitudinal (T1) relaxation so that the next 90° pulse will produce maximum transverse magnetisation. If the TR is short, incomplete relaxation will have taken place and only a corresponding proportion of transverse magnetisation will be produced by the next RF pulse. Therefore, it follows that **signal increases with increasing TR** (Figure 3.1).

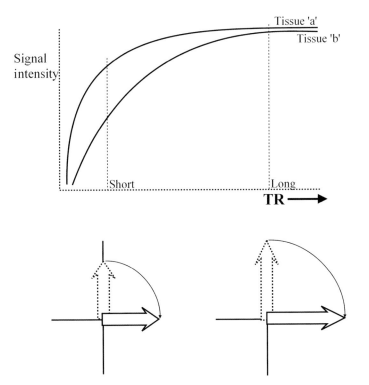

Figure 3.1 The effect of TR on longitudinal magnetisation. How much magnetisation is flipped into the transverse plane is dependent on how much recovered in the longitudinal plane. This increases with TR.

Echo time

Similarly, the longer we wait to collect an echo, the more dephasing of magnetic moments has taken place in the transverse plane. Transverse (T2) relaxation leads to a decrease in signal. So **signal decreases with longer TE** (Figure 3.2).

Flip angle

In gradient echo sequences flip angle will determine the amount of transverse magnetisation, 90° being maximum and giving most signal. Smaller flip angles such as those required for T2* weighting (15–25°) will have **a smaller transverse component and, therefore, less signal**. (Figure 3.3).

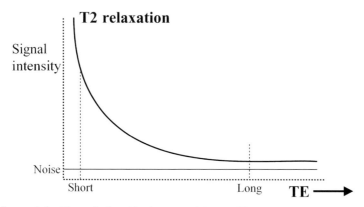

Figure 3.2 The relationship between TE and T2 relaxation.

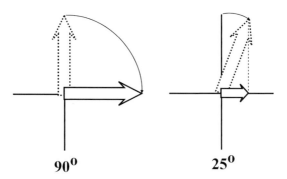

Figure 3.3 Smaller flip angles result in less transverse magnetisation.

Matrix and field of view

The number of phase and frequency encoding steps chosen determines the image matrix size. The field of view (FOV) determines how much anatomy is included in the image. Dividing FOV by matrix will give the pixel size, e.g. a 25 cm FOV with a 256 × 256 matrix will give pixels of (approximately) 1 mm × 1 mm. Since pixels are the elements that make up the image, their size will determine the **area resolution** of the image, hence, the smaller the pixels the better the resolution. Pixel size can be decreased by increasing the number of encoding steps or by decreasing the FOV, or by using a combination of both. Unfortunately, however, the pixel size also determines how much tissue and, in turn, how many protons each pixel represents. Since it is hydrogen that produces signal, it follows that **in decreasing pixel size we not only improve resolution but we decrease SNR since fewer hydrogen spins are included in each pixel** (Figure 3.4).

Slice thickness

Although MR images are two dimensional, they represent a three-dimensional volume of tissue. This third dimension is determined by the slice thickness. The three-dimensional picture element is

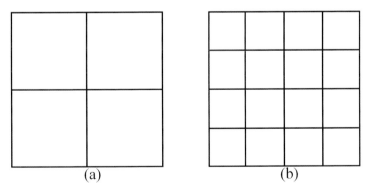

(a)   (b)

Figure 3.4 A summary of the relationship between matrix size, area resolution, SNR and scan time. Each matrix has the same FOV but (b) has twice as many encoding steps. (a) has poorer resolution but better SNR; (b) has better resolution but poorer SNR; (b) takes twice as long to acquire as (a).

described as a voxel, the volume of which is given as pixel area × slice thickness. Again the voxel volume will determine the number of hydrogen spins contributing signal so that, for a given area resolution, **as slice thickness increases so too does SNR**.

Slice thickness, whilst not having an impact on area resolution (remember this is dependent upon pixel size), does determine **spatial resolution** since this takes into account the ability to resolve structures within the slice. The signal from a very small structure within a relatively thick slice will be averaged out at image reconstruction and will effectively disappear. (See Chapter 4 for more about this phenomenon.)

Signal averages

Referred to by manufacturers as 'number of excitations (NEX)' [IGE], 'number of acquisitions' [Siemens], 'number of signal averages (NSA)' [Philips], this represents the number of times each phase encoding step is sampled. Doing this more than once increases SNR, not by increasing the amount of signal received but by reducing the amount of noise sampled since the noise element is random and can therefore be averaged out. This **improvement in SNR is proportional to the square root of the number of samples** as shown in Figure 3.5.

Performing two signal averages instead of one whilst increasing SNR by 40% will, of course, take twice as long. Remember:

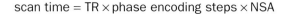

$$\text{scan time} = TR \times \text{phase encoding steps} \times NSA$$

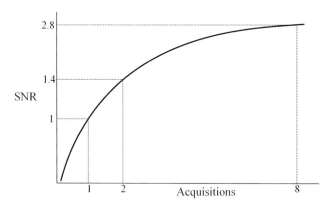

Figure 3.5 The relationship between NSA and signal to noise ratio.

Receive bandwidth

This refers to the range of radiofrequencies sampled at readout. Sampling a smaller range will improve SNR since less noise, which occurs at all frequencies, will be collected. Selecting a narrow bandwidth, however, increases chemical shift artefact (see Chapter 4) and takes longer to sample so may have an impact, indirectly, on scan time.

Device parameters

The only device that the operator has any control over on a day-to-day basis is the choice of receiver coil. This can dramatically improve SNR as described in Chapter 2.

It should be remembered that the amount of signal available is determined by the patient's tissue parameters so choice of coils will not increase the amount of signal available but, in the example in Figure 2.3, using a smaller coil reduces the amount of noise collected, thereby increasing SNR.

Contrast

Contrast is the mechanism in image quality, which allows differentiation of the various tissues according to their signal intensities. This differentiation becomes apparent in the image as different shades of grey and it is the superior soft tissue differentiation of MRI that sets it apart from other imaging techniques. Image contrast is covered in the section on image weighting but, briefly, is dependent on the choice of pulse sequence, imaging parameters and the use (or otherwise) of contrast agents. From earlier discussions in this chapter, it can be seen that choosing a long TR and a short TE would both be options to give the maximum amount of signal. However, the discussion on image weighting indicates that this combination will make the resultant image proton density weighted, giving poorer contrast than T1 or T2 weighting: yet another trade-off.

Artefacts

An artefact is a signal intensity in the image which does not correspond either physically or in spatial distribution to tissues in the imaging slice. The causes of various artefacts, along with various strategies for artefact reduction, are covered extensively in Chapter 4 but the major causes are:

- physiological motion – respiration, flow, peristalsis, patient movement etc.;
- chemical shift;
- susceptibility – caused by the presence of metal or other non-magnetisable material in or near the imaging volume;
- system induced.

4 Image Artefacts: Recognition and Reduction

In Chapter 3, an artefact was defined as a signal intensity in the image which does not correspond, either physically or in spatial distribution, to tissues in the imaging slice. In other words the final image shows an area of signal which has either arisen accidentally or has been displayed in the wrong place. Improvements in equipment and software design over the years have meant that erroneous signal artefacts are becoming increasingly rare. Problems with patient movement are still very much the most common cause of image artefacts. Even anaesthetised animals present problems; physiological motion arising from respiration, blood flow, heartbeat, peristalsis etc. can all lead to misregistration of signal in the final image. This chapter looks at the common causes of image artefacts and at how manufacturers and operators take steps to deal with them.

Movement artefact

Descriptions of spatial encoding, in Chapter 1, showed that encoding in the phase direction involves repeated applications of varying phase encoding gradients throughout the scan acquisition. Application of the frequency encoding gradient, on the other hand, occurs momentarily as the signal or echo is read. It follows then that motion-related artefacts will occur in the phase encoding direction due to the movement of protons between the applications of each phase encoding gradient and that of the readout gradient.

Figure 4.1 shows a diagrammatic representation of flowing blood passing through the imaging slice. Protons arriving in the imaging slice from outside the volume of excitation will not have received any RF energy and will show a complete absence of signal or 'signal void' but protons arriving from an adjacent imaging slice will have been excited but will have the wrong phase for their particular geographical location and will, consequently, be displayed in the wrong place in the image (Figure 4.2). Such artefacts will always be propagated in the phase encoding direction, so an easy way of dealing with them is to swap phase and frequency

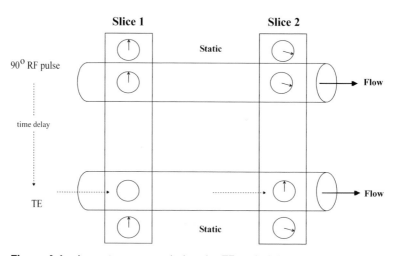

Figure 4.1 As protons move during the TE period they show inappropriate phase at the time of readout.

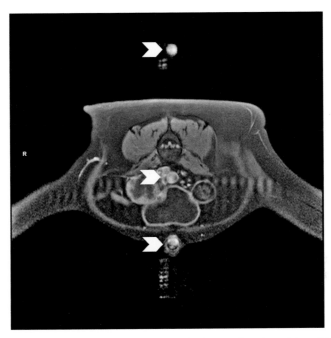

Figure 4.2 Flowing blood in the abdominal aorta is misregistered in the image (arrowheads).

directions. Whilst this will not eliminate the artefact, it will make it run in the other direction through the image so that superimposition over essential structures can be avoided. A good example occurs in transverse imaging of the spine where artefact from aortic pulsation will be propagated directly across the spinal canal if phase runs in the dorsal to ventral direction but, harmlessly, across the abdomen if the phase encoding direction is switched to left–right.

Another way the operator can minimise movement artefact is to increase the number of signal averages (NSA). Since movement tends to be random and signal reproducible, the more each phase encoding step is averaged, the lower will be the impact of movement artefact. The downside of this remedy is that increasing NSA will also increase scan time.

Other available methods of reducing motion artefact are provided by manufacturers and will depend on the type of equipment in use. Some low field systems being marketed for veterinary use are, in fact, designed for imaging human extremities (knee, wrist, ankle etc.) where motion is hardly an issue. Consequently such systems currently offer no facilities for motion artefact reduction. More sophisticated, high field systems, however, tackle motion artefact in one or more of three methods: compensation, gating or presaturation.

Compensation

Movement compensation techniques are many and their exact mechanism will vary from one equipment manufacturer to another; the reader is advised to consult their manufacturer's documentation for precise details. In broad terms, however, respiratory compensation will involve the use of some sort of bellows device to record the pattern of respiration. The scanner will then use this information to reorder phase encoding steps so that the movement between each relative to the respiration curve is minimal, thus reducing phase mismapping. Alternatively some systems will deliberately maximize mismapping so that artefacts are projected as far away as possible from the region of interest.

Other methods of flow compensation use gradient coils in an attempt to correct phase shift in moving protons. This can be effective in slow flow such as that encountered in cerebrospinal fluid and venous blood. Again the exact mechanism will vary with equipment manufacturer.

Gating

A particularly effective way of eliminating motion artefact is to use some form of physiological gating or triggering. In the case of respiration movement, the same bellows device mentioned earlier is used to record the animal's respiration curve. At the point of expiration the MR system is triggered to collect a phase encoding step for each slice being obtained. The system will then stop and wait for the next expiration to trigger another data acquisition. Consequently data are obtained during expiration

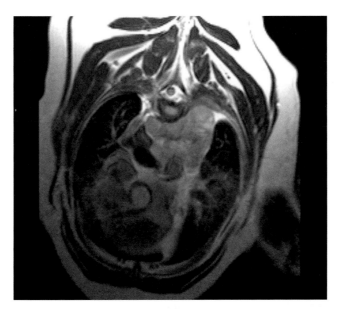

Figure 4.3 T2 weighted transverse image acquired using respiratory gating.

whilst least movement is taking place. This works particularly well in dogs where most animals show a period of long stable expiration punctuated by short, steep intakes of breath. The technique falls short somewhat when the patient is panting or breathing erratically.

It should be noted that repetition time (TR) is now being determined by the patient's respiration rate and will, inevitably, be long. Respiratory triggering, therefore, is most suited to T2 weighted sequences (Figure 4.3). Note that the T1 weighted image (Figure 4.4), obtained without using respiratory gating, shows significant motion artefact from the chest wall. Attempting to obtain T1 weighted images using respiratory gating will invariably result in PD weighting because of the increased TR.

Presaturation

A presaturation pulse is a 90° RF pulse applied to tissue either outside or within the imaging field of view (but not, of course, over

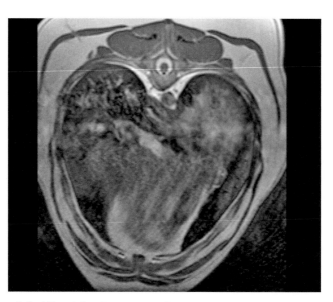

Figure 4.4 T1 weighted transverse image acquired without gating. Note the considerable artefact due to respiratory motion.

the region of interest), just before the 90° excitation pulse is applied. Such tissue will, consequently, receive a total 180° RF excitation and will, therefore, have no transverse component. The result is that this tissue will produce a signal void in the image. If the tissue selected was subject to movement; flowing blood, abdominal wall movement, etc. then a signal void is produced rather than artefact.

Multiple presaturation pulses can be used in combination, for example cranial and caudal to a stack of transverse slices to saturate flowing protons in arterial and venous blood. These are RF pulses, however and, as such, will increase the RF heating effect and can increase scan time. In light of this they should only be used appropriately.

Phase wrap or aliasing

Another common problem closely associated with phase encoding is phase wrap, sometimes also referred to as aliasing or wrap around. To understand why this occurs it should be borne in mind that, in MRI, there are advantages in using a rectangular field of view. By making the short side of the rectangle the phase encoding direction, a rectangular FOV can reduce scan time since there are fewer phase encoding steps. This is particularly suitable where the anatomical area being examined will fit into a rectangular image such as the sagittal spine.

Problems occur, however, when the anatomy being examined does not fit into the field of view. If a field of view is chosen that is too small to encompass the whole of the anatomy in question, the parts left outside will still produce signal. In order to properly map phase signals, the whole phase cycle (0–360°) must be sampled within a given field of view. Where anatomy exists outside this range of samples, duplication of phase positions will occur since it is not possible to go beyond 360° without arriving back at 0. In practice this means that two areas of anatomy will be displayed in the same part of the image (Figure 4.5) with the danger that a lesion could be obscured or a lesion falsely interpreted where none exists.

Increasing FOV so that it encompasses all of the anatomy will, of course, avoid the problem of phase wrap but will also sacrifice image resolution. Image resolution can be maintained by increas-

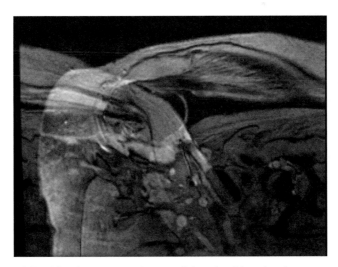

Figure 4.5   T2*W transverse image of the shoulder showing gross artefact caused by wrapping round of anatomy not included in the field of view.

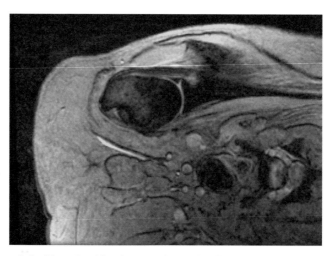

Figure 4.6 The shoulder image shown in Figure 4.5 this time using 'foldover suppression' to eliminate artefact.

Table 4.1 Foldover suppression: the actions involved and the consequential effects on image quality and scan time.

Action	Consequence
FOV is doubled	Anatomy is included
	Resolution decreases
	SNR increases
Phase encoding steps doubled	Resolution increases; returns to original
	Scan time doubles
NSA halved	SNR decreases; returns to original
	Scan time halves; returns to original

ing the number of phase encoding steps but this, in turn, leads to an increase in scan time. However, because the increased number of phase encoding steps also results in an increased SNR, the number of signal averages can be reduced to reduce scan time. If this all sounds very complicated, the good news is that most manufacturers enable all these changes automatically by selecting a single option. GE calls this 'no phase wrap' whilst the Phillips term is 'foldover suppression'. Table 4.1 summarises the various actions that happen when this imaging option is selected and the consequence of each step on image quality.

This combination of changes eliminates aliasing artefact (Figure 4.6) with no apparent compromise of image quality. In practice there may be some detriment due to movement since the reduced number of signal averages fails to average out errors due to movement.

Frequency wrap

Undersampling in the frequency direction can, theoretically, lead to a similar wrapping round of the image in this direction. Most modern MRI systems are so robust in their design that they do not allow this to happen and operators are highly unlikely to encounter this phenomenon.

Chemical shift

Hydrogen exists within the body either in combination with oxygen, as water, or with carbon, as fat. In these combinations hydrogen precesses at slightly different frequencies due to molecular binding effects. The precessional frequency of fat is slightly lower than that of water. It is this variation in precessional frequency that gives rise to the phenomenon of chemical shift.

Since the variation in precessional frequency is proportional to main magnetic field strength (B_0), the chemical shift artefact becomes more pronounced in high field systems. At 1.0 T fat and water precess 147 Hz apart whilst at 1.5 T the difference is 220 Hz. In low field permanent magnet systems of 0.2 T or less the difference is virtually insignificant.

The frequency encoding gradient will establish a range of frequencies across the FOV, and the readout process needs to sample not just a single frequency but this range or bandwidth of frequencies. This is referred to as the receive bandwidth. Dividing the receive bandwidth by the number of frequency encoding steps will give the range of frequencies represented in each pixel. For example, given a 256 matrix with a receive bandwidth of 25 KHz, then each pixel in the final image will represent protons within a prcessional frequency range of approximately 100 Hz. At 1.5 T

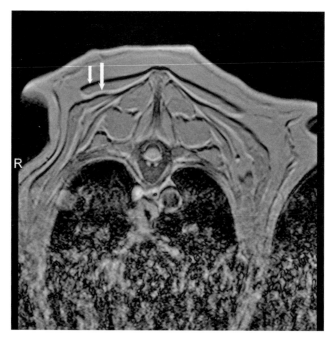

Figure 4.7 Chemical shift artefact is characterised by black and white lines (arrowed) at tissue interfaces.

adjacent fat and water molecules in the patient (which have a frequency difference of 220 Hz) will be displayed two pixels apart. If the FOV is 25 cm this will represent a difference in the image of roughly 2 mm (25 cm ÷ 256). The resultant image shows a 2 mm line each side (black one side, white the other) of structures which have a fat/water or fat/tissue interface, e.g. bladder, intervertebral discs, kidneys, muscle etc. (Figure 4.7).

The way to reduce chemical shift artefact is to use a larger receive bandwidth. In the example above for instance, using a receive bandwidth of 50 KHz would reduce the artefact to only 1 mm. The downside, however, is that using a larger receive bandwidth also causes a reduction in SNR (see Chapter 3).

Do not be surprised to find that receive bandwidth is not an obviously selectable parameter on all MR systems. Siemens include bandwidth as part of a selectable sequence file whilst

Philips disguise it as 'fat/water shift'; selecting maximum fat/ water shift is, in practical terms, the same as selecting the smallest available receive bandwidth. Only GE displays receive bandwidth as a clearly separate selectable parameter. In low field systems, where chemical shift is not an issue, the operator will have no control over receive bandwidth.

Chemical misregistration

The difference in precessional frequency between fat and water leads to another phenomenon which can give rise to image artefacts. Consider the paths of two protons precessing at slightly different frequencies (Figure 4.8). For most of the time they will be out of phase with each other but at a certain point on their path they will be perfectly in phase. Try thinking of them as the two hands of a clock which, at certain times of day, will be superimposed: 12 o'clock for example.

Likewise, at certain points on their paths the magnetic moments of these two protons will oppose each other. At points where fat and water are in phase with each other their signals will combine, whilst at points where they are opposed they will cancel each other out. Pixels in the image which contain fat and water (particularly in equal amounts) will go through instances of maximum signal (fat and water in phase) and signal void (fat and water opposed). If TE is selected to coincide with one or other of these conditions, the same point in the image could be made to look bright (in phase) or dark (out of phase). In spin echo

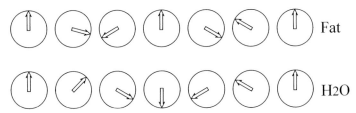

Figure 4.8   Fat and water precess at slightly different frequencies.

sequences this problem is, largely, eliminated by the 180° refocusing pulse, but in gradient echo sequences it is exaggerated. Selecting a TE which coincides with the out of phase condition in gradient echo sequences can result in a black line in the image at fat/water interfaces, e.g. around the kidneys. Some radiologists find this strange appearance useful in certain instances such as imaging of the adrenal glands. In most instances, however, it can be avoided by selecting the 'in phase' option as the TE parameter (most systems will then calculate the correct echo time automatically).

Susceptibility artefact

Sometimes referred to as metallic artefact, since metal is often the cause, susceptibility describes the ability of a substance to become magnetized. Susceptibility artefact occurs at interfaces between substances with very diverse susceptibility. Metal is the obvious cause but air is also a culprit and susceptibility artefact is sometimes seen in the region of the frontal sinuses, particularly in breeds where the sinuses are large.

The 180° refocusing pulse found in spin echo sequences goes some way to compensating for the phase shift brought about by susceptibility. Consequently fast or turbo spin echo sequences with their multiple 180° RF pulses produce the least artefact whilst gradient echo sequences that do not employ RF to refocus spins, produce the most severe artefact.

In animals the most common example of such an artefact is that produced on images of the neck by ID chips (Figure 4.9). Another example is provided by the small coiled springs found in the cuff valves of some endotracheal tubes; care should be taken to keep the valve out of the FOV.

To reduce the impact of such artefacts all metallic objects, including those that are non-ferromagnetic, should be removed wherever possible. There are even rare cases when removal of an ID chip may have to be considered. Where metalwork is firmly implanted, fast spin echo sequences should be favoured to keep distortion to a minimum.

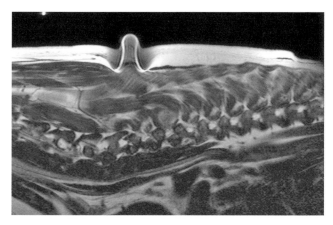

Figure 4.9   Susceptibility artefact from ID chip.

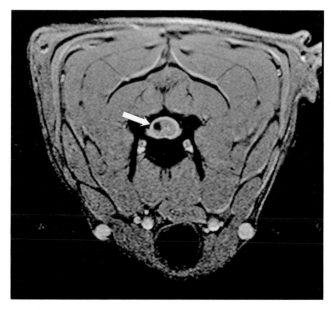

Figure 4.10   Cervical spinal cord haemorrhage giving rise to susceptibility artefact on T2 gradient echo sequence.

Susceptibility artefact can be used to advantage in cases where old haemorrhage is suspected. One of the breakdown products of blood is haemosiderin which has a high iron content. On gradient echo sequences, in particular, haemosiderin causes a marked susceptibility effect (Figure 4.10).

System-induced artefacts

These are artefacts that arise as a result of some sort of error or malfunction of the MR system itself. Invariably their correction will involve the assistance of the service engineer. Figure 4.11, for example, shows the artefact produced by a voltage surge during scanning: a so-called electrical spike. Just occasionally, however, the remedy can be a simple one. The 'zipper' artefact, for example, is caused by erroneous RF signal being picked up by the receiver coil and incorporated into the image (Figure 4.12). This can mean a defect in the scan room's Faraday cage or may be corrected simply by making sure the scan room door remains firmly closed during scanning. Faulty light bulbs are also a common source of RF transmissions. Make sure blown or flickering lights in the scan room are replaced. Note that the 'zipper' occurs along the frequency direction at a position determined by the frequency of the stray signal.

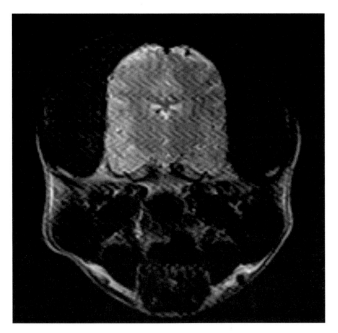

Figure 4.11 Artefact caused by voltage surge during acquisition.

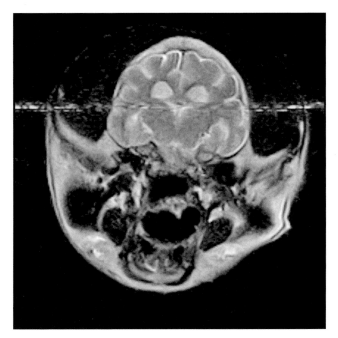

Figure 4.12 Zipper artefact caused by RF interference.

Partial volume averaging

Finally a word about 'partial volume averaging'. Although not, strictly speaking, an artefact, this phenomenon can often lead to image misinterpretation or failure to demonstrate small lesions.

Partial volume averaging describes how the MR system handles signal arising from anatomical structures which fail to fully fill the imaging slice in the slice selection direction (the slice thickness). Figure 4.13 shows a simplified representation of two adjacent structures, one white and one black. The imaging slice has been prescribed such that it is filled equally by both structures. When signal intensity is measured by the system it will detect 50% white and 50% black. The resultant image will demonstrate neither a black or white structure but a grey one. It could be argued that

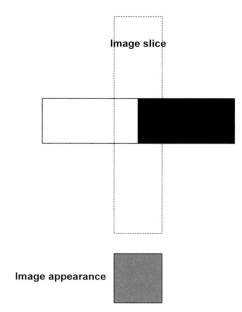

Figure 4.13 Different signal intensities occuring within the same slice thickness are averaged.

this gives rise to an artefact since no grey structure exists but, at the same time, it is a true representation of the net signal intensity within the selected slice.

Now consider the same area scanned with two imaging slices each of half the thickness (Figure 4.14). In this example our black and white structures each occupy a complete (thinner) slice. The resultant images will display these structures as black on one image and white on the other. Spatial resolution (as discussed in chapter 3) has been improved allowing more accurate demonstration of the structures under examination.

This example is obviously very simplified for explanatory reasons but in the clinical setting it is important to bear in mind that there are two major pitfalls that may result from the way anatomy is resolved in the slice thickness direction. One is that very small structures or lesions can be missed in sections that are too thick and the other is that false lesions can be inferred which are, in

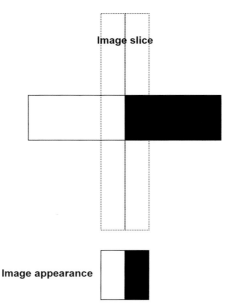

Figure 4.14 Using thinner sections allows accurate representation of each signal intensity.

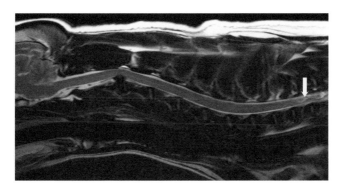

Figure 4.15 Apparent high signal within the spinal cord is, in fact, caused by adjacent epidural fat.

fact, encroachment of adjacent (usually high signal) tissues. This is a common pitfall in parasagittal images of the spinal cord (low signal) where it lies in contact with epidural fat (high signal) (Figure 4.15).

PART TWO
MRI in Veterinary Practice

5 MRI Safety

Magnets and magnetic fields

The MRI systems most often encountered in veterinary practice employ either permanent or superconducting magnets. Except in emergency situations, neither of these magnet types can be switched off; consequently **the magnetic field is always on** even when the rest of the imaging system is shut down. Superconducting magnets can be shut down in an emergency situation by activating the emergency off mechanism which rapidly 'boils off' the liquid helium reducing the field to zero in a matter of minutes, a process known as 'quenching' the magnet. This is a very costly exercise due to the price of liquid helium and the expense of refilling and re-energizing the magnet; it should not be undertaken lightly.

Magnetic field strength is measured in units called Gauss (G) or Tesla (T); $10000\,G = 1\,T$. Magnetic fields in excess of $5\,G$ can adversely affect cardiac pacemakers with potentially fatal consequences. For this reason all areas where personnel may encounter magnetic fields over $5\,G$ are designated as **controlled areas**. In practice this, more often than not, means the same room as the scanner itself. Even at $1.5\,T$ the $5\,G$ line is usually contained within the scan room.

Safety issues

MRI has been used extensively in human medicine for many years now and is becoming increasingly common in veterinary practice. There are no known side effects and the procedure is regarded as safe for patients and operators alike. However, because of the very strong magnetic field involved there are a number of extremely important safety issues, which must be understood, particularly by those entering the controlled area.

The Medical Devices Agency (MDA) identified three main hazards associated with MRI, namely: the static magnetic field, B_0; time-varying magnetic field gradients; and radiofrequency (RF) magnetic fields (B_1).

The static magnetic field, B_0

There are several areas of concern relating to the static magnetic field. Perhaps most important is the so-called projectile effect but also worthy of consideration are the biological effects, and the safety and compatibility of implanted devices and ancillary equipment, such as patient monitoring devices. Magnets employed in clinical veterinary use range from 0.2–1.5 T. Even at the lower end of this range, these magnets are powerful enough to attract loose ferro-magnetic objects and accelerate them towards the centre of the magnet bore, causing significant damage to anyone or anything getting in the way. Consequently no ferro-magnetic materials should be allowed into the scan room. This means that animals should have collars etc. removed and all personnel should remove metallic objects (pens, scissors, coins etc.) before entering the scan room. The wearing of 'white coats' in the MRI area is discouraged as these represent an excellent hiding place for assorted metallic hardware.

Although experiments with primates carried out at field strengths above 4–5 T suggested cardiac arrhythmia and reduced mental function, a 1991 report from the National Radiological Board (NRPB) concludes that magnetic fields of less than 2.5 T are unlikely to have any detrimental effect on health.

Despite there being no adverse biological effects from the static magnetic field, certain implanted medical devices can be affected. Such devices include stents, clips, neurostimulators and, in particular, cardiac pacemakers. Pacemakers can be adversely affected by fields as low as 1 mT. Not only should patients with such devices be excluded (there are a number of dogs with cardiac pacemakers) but staff with these implants should not be allowed into the scan room either.

To avoid the introduction of potentially dangerous materials into the controlled area, each practice involved in MRI should set out a system of practice or local rules to govern who is authorised to enter the controlled area and ensure that they are adequately prepared and screened for potential hazards. Warning signs should be displayed at the entry to the controlled area advising of the dangers posed by the high magnetic field (Figure 5.1).

It should be noted that surgical implants made from high-grade stainless or surgical steel or titanium are non-ferrous and as such will not be attracted by the magnet. Significant susceptibility artefact will be caused (less so in the case of titanium) when such implants are in or near the field of view.

Time-varying magnetic fields – gradients

Many of the functions discussed in Chapter 1 (spatial localisation, slice location, frequency encoding etc.) rely on the three time-varying magnetic fields or gradients, gx, gy and gz. These are supplementary magnetic fields generated by gradient coils that are switched on and off very rapidly.

Unlike B_0, these are changing magnetic fields and as such are capable of inducing a current in a suitable electrical conductor. It is very important to make sure no such conductors are introduced into the bore of the magnet where induced currents could cause the conductor to heat up and burn the patient. Particular problems can occur with monitoring leads. If wire leads are allowed to form a loop then a current can be induced causing the wire to heat. Care should be taken to ensure that all leads used for monitoring, physiological gating, RF coils etc. are kept straight and separated from the patient, particularly in short-haired breeds.

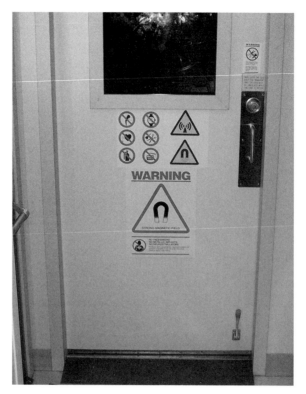

Figure 5.1 The scan room door should carry a suitable sign warning of the strong magnetic field.

New MR systems have very fast, and strong, gradients capable of rates of change in the order of 25–30 mT/m in 0.5–1.0 mS. These can stimulate nerve or muscle fibres and have the potential to cause ventricular fibrillation, epileptogenic effects, visual flash sensations and the like. This sort of side effect is not very likely during routine clinical investigations but ultra-fast scanning techniques like echo planar imaging must be used with some care.

Radiofrequency energy deposition

Whilst not ionising radiation, the radiofrequency used in MRI is, nonetheless, electromagnetic radiation and, as such, deposits its energy, in the form of heat, in the patient's body. This is then dissipated and removed by conduction, convection and radiation and is, therefore, dependent on many physiological, physical and environmental factors such as ambient temperature, humidity, airflow, coat thickness, the patient's physiological state and so on. All these factors limit the rate at which heat is lost from the body. The rate at which heat is being deposited is, therefore, critical to avoid simulating a microwave oven!

Specific absorption rate

The rate of heat deposition is indicated by the specific absorption rate (SAR). For a given pulse sequence it is dependent on the duration, amplitude and number of RF pulses (including presaturation pulses) during each TR. SAR is measured in Watts per kilogram for whole body exposure. Most clinical MR examinations will have SARs of less than 0.4 W/kg but some newer sequences such as fast spin echo can reach 2.0 W/Kg. Particularly sensitive organs are the eyes and testes. For a homogeneous sphere of tissue (like those *never* encountered in the animal body!) of radius **r**; conductivity σ; in a magnetic field $\mathbf{B_o}$, SAR is proportional to the flip angle α thus:

$$\mathbf{SAR} \propto \sigma \mathbf{r}^2 \mathbf{B_o^2} \alpha^2 \mathbf{D}$$

where **D** is the duty cycle, i.e. the percentage of time during the sequence for which RF is applied. The good news is that SAR is calculated automatically by scanner software. Auto-sensing circuits use details of the patient's weight along with the factors for the particular sequence to calculate the SAR and prevent the scan if the SAR is too high. No attempts should be made to bypass this safety feature. The solution is to reduce the RF energy being used, e.g. by reducing the number of slices, or increase the time frame by increasing TR. The temptation to guess or lie about the patient's weight should be resisted.

Whilst it is not suggested that you memorise the above formula (hooray!) two points should be noted. Firstly because SAR is proportional to the square of B_0, it rises rapidly with increasing field strength. This means that SAR limits are more of a problem at

1.5 T than 0.5 T. Similarly, because SAR is also proportional to the square of the flip angle, 180° pulses deposit four times as much energy as do 90° pulses. This means that sequences such as fast spin echo, with multiple 180° pulses, generate much more heat than low flip angle, gradient echo sequences.

Acoustic noise

It can't have escaped the attention of anyone who has experienced an MR scan just how noisy the technique can be. Increase in current in gradient coils is opposed by the static field and generates noise. The effect is proportional to B_0 and therefore is greater in high field systems. Levels of up to 105 dB have been recorded and temporary reduction of hearing has been reported in some patients following a scan. Whilst it is difficult to provide effective hearing protection for animals, it is advisable to provide earplugs or some other form of ear protection for personnel who need to be present in the scan room during MR examinations, particularly on higher field systems with powerful gradients.

Further reading

This chapter gives an overview of the major safety concerns relating to MRI. Undoubtedly the best source of safety information is the equipment manufacturer's manual. This will cover some of the topics above as well as matters relating specifically to the equipment in question, to cryogens, fire risk, quenching of the system, etc. Reference should also be made to the various publications of the Radiological Protection Board, The Department of Health, Medical Devices Agency (formally MDA, now MHRA) and the local rules.

6 Using MRI in Clinical Veterinary Practice

Introduction

The last 20 years have seen enormous advancements in veterinary imaging. Radiography has been readily available to the veterinary profession for 60 years and recently technical advancements have paralleled the computer revolution. Dry processing machines have removed the need for darkrooms and produce developed, ready-dried X-ray films within minutes. Now digital radiography is available, giving high-resolution images on visual display units and allowing the images to be networked and stored electronically.

Ultrasonography has progressed to the development of sophisticated machines that have increasing application in veterinary practice. Only the cost of the equipment delayed veterinary science from keeping up with medical science in the use of CT and MRI. However, the use of mobile scanners has meant that the throughput needed to justify costs is attainable by visiting many different locations on a regular, rotating basis. Recently high-quality low field MRI scanners have become available. The permanent magnets in these machines, whilst having a strength well below that of the helium-cooled superconducting magnets, yield excellent results. The added advantages of the smaller static scanners are relative ease of operation and the ready availability for scanning patients, e.g. out of normal hours.

Notwithstanding these developments in technology, a CT or MRI scanner is still a large capital investment for general veterinary practice and it is likely that it will be some time before they are purchased by other than large private referral centres and veterinary schools. Perhaps this is not a bad thing since it automatically ensures a quality assurance for clients and insurance companies.

The clarity and quality of the images produced by the MRI scanner do tempt users to employ scanning when it is not truly indicated and also to expect positive results where a full diagnostic work-up would show that a visible lesion is unlikely. It is therefore imperative that users of MRI understand the true application of this remarkable technique and do not try to replace usual, less sophisticated diagnostic procedures.

MRI undoubtedly has its greatest application in studies of the central nervous system. The radiotransparency of nervous tissue and the inaccessibility of the neuraxis to direct observation, have always made the investigation of CNS disease a particular challenge. Myelography was, for many years, the only technique that produced images allowing a visual assessment of compressive lesions of the spinal cord. Although myelography still has its advocates, it has been superseded by MRI on the grounds of patient risk alone.

A sound and thorough knowledge of anatomy is essential for accurate interpretation of MR images. The ability to read the images in three dimensions is an advantage and in any case a set of scans in at least the three orthogonal planes of orientation will usually be necessary to visualise an abnormality fully. The signalling characteristics of the different tissues and those of pathological change need to be appreciated quite apart from the basic understanding that fat is hyperintense and water is hypointense on T1 scans whereas both fat and water are hyperintense on T2 weighted scans. The varying uptake of a contrast agent, like gadolinium, can be very informative about the possible identity of pathological change but it has to be understood that some very vascular normal tissues may also show enhancement with the contrast agent.

Anaesthesia

No painful stimuli result from MRI investigations. All that is required, in terms of anaesthesia or sedation, for a successful examination is that the animal remains still throughout the procedure. As a consequence, the level of anaesthesia required is perhaps less than that required for surgery though some MRI systems can be quite noisy, particularly at high field strength; this will also be a factor in determining the optimum level of sedation/anaesthesia.

Anaesthesia for MRI scanning becomes complicated only because it must be carried out in close proximity to a powerful magnetic field and the rules about magnetically sensitive objects and potential missiles obviously apply. Monitoring of the anaesthetised patient is also made difficult in such an environment. Many of the monitoring devices normally used during anaesthesia simply don't work in proximity to a high magnetic field. This can be overcome by using specialist MRI-compatible monitoring equipment, though this is often very expensive. A cheaper alternative is to modify existing equipment to allow it to be used at a safe distance from the magnet. A capnograph, for instance, can be used outside the scan room simply by extending the sampling line to the patient and passing this through a wave guide (see Figure 2.5). Similarly, oxygen cylinders and other non-MRI-compatible equipment can be kept at a safe distance from the field by using extended tubing. The exact protocol for anaesthesia will, of course, vary according to the preference of the anaesthetist and clinical condition of the patient.

Whereas full anaesthesia is obviously desirable, particularly when the scanning procedure is likely to take more than 15 minutes, heavy sedation can be quite adequate for short procedures. The combination of medetomidine and butorphanol gives a good level of sedation which is quite suitable when the procedure is being carried out for basic screening or routine monitoring (see below). Whether anaesthesia or sedation is being employed, it is important that a physical examination precedes the procedure. There are also good arguments for carrying out haematological and blood biochemical analysis before scanning. A laboratory work-up is likely to be needed for the purposes of diagnosis, but the results may have some significance for the anaesthesia protocol and may indicate caution in the use of a contrast agent, e.g. the existence of severe renal disease. The fact that many of the patients have brain disease and may already be receiving therapy, e.g. anticonvulsants, may influence the choice of anaesthetic drugs. Acepromazine may be used as a premedicant sedative in spinal patients but should be avoided in any patient in which seizures may occur since this drug is known to act as a potential trigger.

It is beyond the scope of this book to discuss different anaesthetic agents and protocols. The usual regime employed by the authors' anaesthetist colleagues is an intravenous induction with propofol followed by gaseous maintenance using isoflurane or sevoflurane.

The combination of medetomidine and butorphanol is ideal for short studies in dogs. The recommended dosages are those for induction of deep sedation; 0.025 ml/kg of a 1 mg/ml solution of medetomidine and 0.01 ml/kg of a 10 mg/ml solution of butorphanol. The two drugs can be administered together in the same syringe by intramuscular or intravenous injection. Generally a period of 15 minutes is required after administration before starting to scan. On completion of scanning the sedation can be reversed by using an equal volume of atipamezole to that of medetomidine used. Recovery to standing is usually within 10 minutes.

Although medetomidine alone or combined with butorphanol and ketamine may be used in cats to obtain deep sedation, the authors prefer general anaesthesia when scanning this species.

Patient positioning

All MR systems available for small animal veterinary use, including those marketed specifically as veterinary systems, have been designed for scanning humans either as whole body scanners or for extremity, muscloskeletal use. As a consequence, scanning animals requires some ingenuity in terms of positioning and choice of coils on the part of the operator. The human knee coil supplied with the low field system shown in Figure 6.1, for example, lends itself nicely to scanning animal brains in sternal recumbency as shown. The design of the high field system head coil shown in

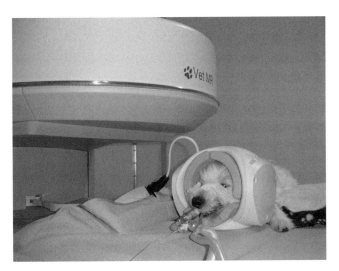

Figure 6.1 Patient positioned in sternal recumbency using an extremity coil.

Figure 6.2, however, is such that animals are easier to accommodate in dorsal recumbency. These considerations notwithstanding, there is a number of factors the operator should take into account when positioning patients and coils in order to optimise image quality. The choice of coil is important as this can have a major impact on SNR (see Chapter 3). Generally speaking the coil should be as small as possible, consistent with including the area of anatomy to be examined. Phased array coils, where available, will give improved SNR over standard linear surface coils.

Patients should be positioned as straight as possible on the scan table. Although MRI can easily employ oblique scan planes to compensate for slight obliquity of the patient, it is important, particularly in spinal imaging, that essential structures do not meander in and out of the imaging slice. Figure 6.3 shows examples of good and bad positioning in sagittal imaging of the spine.

When scanning extremities, consideration should be given to the position of the joint or limb within the bore of the magnet. The most homogeneous part of the field is that closest to the isocentre; consequently, better results will be obtained by scanning near the middle of the bore than round the edges. In large dogs in particular, this will often involve offsetting the animal to one side

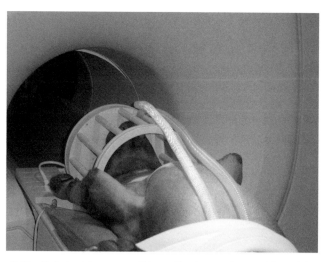

Figure 6.2   Coil design means this patient must be positioned in dorsal recumbency.

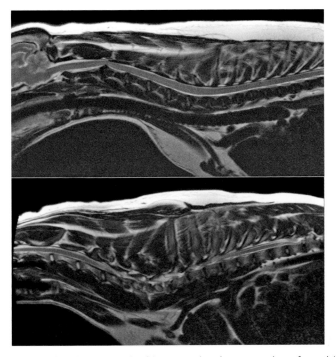

Figure 6.3 T2 weighted sagittal images showing examples of good (top) and poor (lower) patient positioning.

to bring the side under examination into the central part of the magnet. This is especially critical in low field systems where the useable field may be 14 cm or less.

Animals should also be well immobilised so as to prevent movement artefact; even anaesthetised animals can roll to one side if not adequately secured. The use of immobilisation aids such as plastic cradles, sand bags and ties will help achieve this aim. Large, deep-chested breeds such as the Irish wolfhound are particularly difficult to position and require some patience and practice.

Imaging planes

The conventions used in human medicine differ slightly from those used in veterinary imaging. Essentially the three orthogonal planes used in veterinary MRI are sagittal, transverse and dorsal. Since the anatomical position of cats and dogs is standing on all fours, use of the human orthogonal plane coronal can be confusing and is best avoided.

The choice of imaging plane will be determined according to the anatomical area being examined, the clinical findings, the site of pathology and, not least of all, the individual preference of the person interpreting the images. Nevertheless a little thought about the choice of imaging plane and sequences is essential for a quick and effective MRI examination. In spinal studies, for example, it is best to begin with sagittal sections (T2W is most useful) of the clinically indicated area; in smaller animals the whole spine can easily be included. Careful examination of these images will demonstrate any abnormalities, such as a disc prolapse, which need further imaging using transverse oblique sections parallel to the affected disc space(s). These images will help to evaluate the degree of cord compression, nerve root impingement etc. and may well conclude the examination. In conditions such as nerve root tumour, vertebral anomalies and facet joint hypertrophy, however, it may also be beneficial to obtain images in the dorsal plane. In cases where surgical intervention is being considered, dorsal plane imaging can also be helpful in establishing surgical landmarks, as ribs and transitional vertebrae are often better demonstrated in this plane.

One of the major advantages of MRI over other imaging techniques is its ability to image in any plane. The use of a range of oblique planes to supplement the three orthogonal planes can prove an invaluable aid to diagnosis. The indiscriminate use of all three orthogonal planes for each sequence only serves to extend the examination and the anaesthetic unnecessarily.

Contrast agents

The contrast agent used in MRI scanning is usually dimeglumine gadopentetate (gadolinium). This is a paramagnetic contrast medium used in human patients for MRI and for the evaluation of renal function. It is not currently licensed for use in animals but there is no equivalent veterinary licensed product available. This should be understood and noted on the consent form signed by the owner of any animal patient likely to require gadolinium during scanning. Although adverse reactions to gadolinium are rare in dogs and cats, the following should be noted:

- Hypersensitivity reactions may occur with anaphylactoid, cardiovascular and respiratory manifestations. Care must be taken to see that drugs and equipment are available to treat such reactions.
- Seizure disorders: patients suffering from seizures or intracranial lesions may be at increased risk from seizure activity.
- Impaired renal function: gadolinium is excreted renally and careful consideration must be taken before administering the contrast medium to any patient with severe kidney disease.
- Pregnant and very young animals: there are no known special warnings or recorded reactions.

The dose of gadolinium is 0.2 ml/kg administered intravenously and scanning should be commenced immediately. Gadolinium shortens the T1 relaxation time of tissues in which it is present, consequently T1W sequences are used in post-contrast studies.

When examining joints it is often helpful to introduce contrast into the joint fluid to produce 'MR arthrography'. In these instances gadolinium should be diluted in saline at a rate of 1 ml intravenous gadolinium added to 1 litre of saline.

Clinical indications

The current technological advancements, particularly in modern high field MRI systems, mean that the range of clinical applications is extremely diverse. The aim of this section of the book is to provide guidance to the veterinary clinician in helping to obtain the maximum benefit to the patient from the appropriate use of MRI. Much, of course, will depend on the availability of MRI, but also alternative techniques such as ultrasound and CT. The sophistication of the available MRI system will also influence what can be achieved. The clinical applications of an advanced high field system, for example, will far exceed those of a basic low field scanner. Nevertheless, it is hoped that the following guide will help in choosing which patients will benefit from this valuable imaging technique.

The results of MRI scanning can be spectacular and the rapidity with which a diagnosis can be made contrasts with the laborious efforts that sometimes characterised neurology before MRI was available. However, the temptation to scan without a proper physical examination and attention to the history must be resisted. Patients should not be presented for scanning either before a proper physical examination or because the clinician is unable to make a sound clinical analysis of the case. To do so results in frustration and prolonged scanning time, undesirable for both patient and radiographer. Thus it is essential that the clinician tries to localise the lesion as accurately as possible before scanning.

As was the case in human medicine, much MRI imaging time in veterinary medicine is currently devoted to the assessment of the brain and spine but imaging of the musculoskeletal system is already an expanding area of interest amongst orthopaedic specialists. The availability of rapid scanning techniques means that imaging of the soft tissues of the thorax and abdomen will also expand as access to MRI increases and clinical experience grows.

Because of this growth in experience and because MRI is such a rapidly advancing technology, the information presented here should be regarded not as hard and fast rules about what MRI should be used for but as a 'snapshot' of how MRI currently helps to optimise patient care in veterinary practice.

Head

Intracranial lesions

Access to MRI has revolutionised neurology in that it allows imaging of the soft tissue structures within the 'impenetrable box' of the cranium. To be fair, this had already been achieved to a degree by CT but its limited capability in terms of soft tissue differentiation and difficulties of access for the veterinary profession meant that MRI was the truly remarkable breakthrough in brain imaging.

The brain is undoubtedly a very frequent target for MR scanning, not least because direct visualisation and palpation are not possible and radiography is only of limited use. The tissues provide a natural contrast with one another and the cerebrospinal fluid (CSF) helps to 'outline' some of the more easily identified structures. It is helpful, in analysing a lesion and its clinical effects, to consider the brain in six functional regions:

- cerebral hemispheres;
- diencephalon;
- midbrain and pons;
- medulla;
- vestibular;
- cerebellum.

Functional disturbance of each of these regions is usually seen as a characteristic set of clinical signs (Table 6.1). This pre-information before scanning gives some idea of what to expect and assists in the localisation of the lesion. If seizures are due to an intracranial lesion, it is most likely to be located in the

Table 6.1 Some clinical signs of brain lesions in specific regions.

Region of the brain	Clinical signs
Cerebrum	Seizures, behavioural changes, depression, contralateral hemi-paresis, blindness, postural deficits
Diencephalon	Behavioural changes, autonomic signs, postural deficits, blindness
Midbrain/pons	Depression, coma, cranial nerve deficits III–VIII, postural deficits
Medulla	Hemiparesis, ataxia, cranial nerve deficits IX–XII, nystagmus, head tilt
Vestibular	Head tilt, hypertonia, loss of balance, ataxia
Cerebellum	Tremor, dysmetria, ataxia, nystagmus

forebrain or diencephalon. If the seizures include compulsive circling in the postictal or interictal phases then the lesion is most
likely to be on the side to which the circling is directed. With a
few exceptions a head tilt, leaning and loss of balance suggest
that a lesion involves the vestibular pathways and, if central, will
be in the medulla oblongata. So in many circumstances the lesion
will be located where indicated by the clinical signs. The value
of careful assessment of the clinical signs and a competent
neurological examination is realised when the lesion is not so
obvious as it may be. In this situation the use of STIR and FLAIR
procedures or a contrast agent may reward conscientious
localisation.

It is often worth remembering that multiple lesions or diffuse
lesions are not uncommon in the brain. In the cat multiple meningiomas occur frequently (Figure 6.4) and in the dog diffuse inflam-

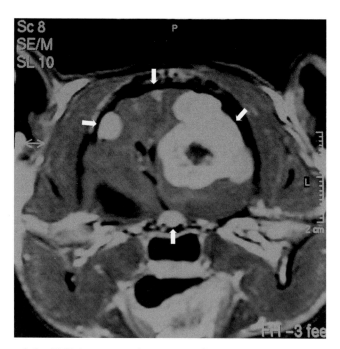

Figure 6.4 T1W transverse image post intravenous contrast showing
multiple meningiomas (arrowed) in a feline patient.

matory disease of the brain is seen regularly, e.g. steroid-responsive encephalitis and granulomatous meningoencephalitis. Focal lesions are usually lateralised, apart from those that involve midline structures like the pituitary gland. Expanding lesions, e.g. neoplasms, are often surrounded by oedema due to disturbance of cell membrane permeability as a result of compression of the tissues. The restriction on expansion by the surrounding skull results in distortion of the tissues, obliteration of the cavities of the ventricles and herniation of tissues caudally. The most frequent distortion due to an expanding space-occupying lesion is a midline shift.

Although some oedema may occur in association with a vascular accident, especially an infarction, swelling rarely is seen. The absence of a midlne shift and limited diffuse hyperintensity on T2W scans help to differentiate vascular lesions from neoplasia.

Neoplasia

The site, size, distribution and often the nature of intracranial tumours are very well demonstrated using MRI. In addition, MRI can give the neurosurgeon valuable information as to the resectability or otherwise of intracranial tumours. Neoplasms grow at varying rates, e.g. meningiomas are slow, taking years to reach a stage when clinical signs are apparent, whereas gliomas are rapid-growing and often out-grow their vascular supply resulting in central necrosis and poor enhancement with gadolinium. Meningiomas are often well circumscribed, indicating good prospects of excision but gliomas often have a 'blurred' outline where the surrounding tissues are infiltrated and the prospects of surgical excision are poor.

Meningiomas are the commonest brain tumours in dogs and cats. They grow inwards from the arachnoid mater and may be calcified or cystic. Quite frequently the MRI scans reveal that the neoplastic tissue extends within the meninges on the surface of the brain to form a plaque. Common sites for meningiomas are the olfactory lobes, within the skull vault (Figure 6.5), the region of the optic chiasma, the cranio-cervical junction (Figure 6.6) and the ventral aspect of the brainstem. Meningiomas usually enhance

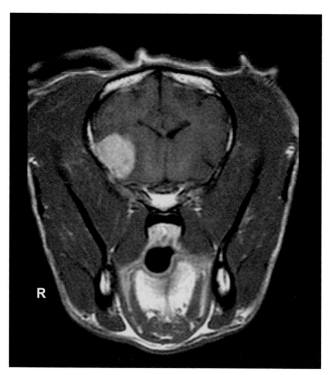

Figure 6.5 T1W transverse image post intravenous contrast showing a meningioma of the right parietal region.

brightly and homogeneously with gadolinium; on T2W there is hyperintensity due to the associated oedema. Gliomas (Figure 6.7) are probably the second most frequent brain tumours in dogs and can occur at a young age. Gliomas may show only poor enhancement with gadolinium and usually are irregular in outline. Gliomas often are hyperintense on T2 weighting, are surrounded by oedema and may possess a necrotic hypointense centre (on T1W). Choroid plexus papillomas and ependymomas are hyperintense on T2W scans and are located around the ventricular system.

The normal pituitary gland enhances with gadolinium and can be quite hyperintense on T2W scans. Since the neoplastic pituitary gland does not necessarily appear enlarged, this can be misleading and emphasises the need for laboratory evidence of endocrine disturbance. However, macroadenomas (Figures 6.8

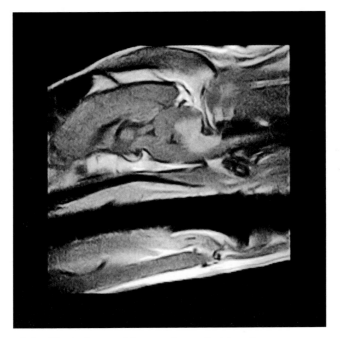

Figure 6.6 Meningioma of the cranio-cervical junction.

and 6.9) are very well demonstrated and can often explain neuro-logical signs such as blindness due to disruption of the optic chiasma. A macroadenoma of the pituitary gland often shows extension into the diencephalon.

Vascular lesions

Cerebrovascular accidents (CVAs) are well recognised in human patients and are called 'strokes'. They are sudden in onset and may be due to either an infarction or a haemorrhage. Clinically they can be catastrophic resulting in hemiplegia, loss of speech, etc. For many years the veterinary literature insisted that 'strokes' did not occur in animals and then the situation became further confused by the frequent use of the term 'stroke' for acute ves-tibular disease. This was a double error in that there was no proof that there had been a vascular accident and it was quite the wrong location, probably even peripheral rather than central.

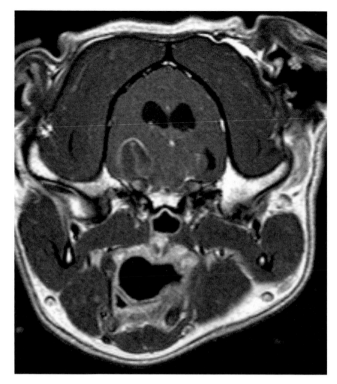

Figure 6.7 Transverse T1W post-contrast study showing patchy enhancement of a probable glioma in the right temporal region.

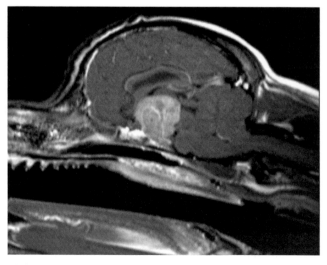

Figure 6.8 Sagittal T1W post-contrast image showing a pituitary tumour.

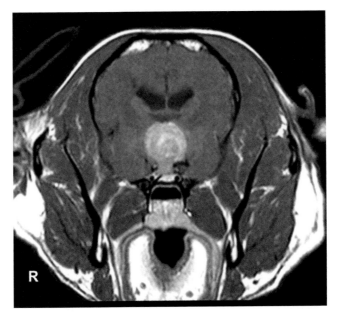

Figure 6.9 The same lesion as Figure 6.8 shown in the transverse plane.

MRI has now shown that spontaneous intracranial vascular accidents do indeed occur in companion animals. Haemorrhage may be intraparenchymal, subarachnoid, subdural or epidural. The exact MRI appearance of haemorrhage is a little difficult to predict since it changes with the breakdown of blood within the clot. Work in human patients has demonstrated the pattern of change summarised in Table 6.2.

Comparative studies have not been carried out in animals and, whilst it seems reasonable to expect a similar pattern of change in MRI appearance, caution must be exercised in applying the same data to other species. Most CVAs that are diagnosed with the help of MRI will be scanned within a few days of onset and so haemorrhages will be focal and bright on T2W. Infarcts are seen as areas of diffuse hyperintensity. Figure 6.10 shows the typical T1W and T2W appearances of a temporal lobe infarction. In either type of vascular accident involving the forebrain, the presenting clinical sign is likely to be a seizure. Whereas vascular

Table 6.2 Changes in MRI signalling characteristics of intracranial haemorrhage.

Time	T1	T2	Biochemistry	Comments
Hyperacute (the first 2–3 h)	Dark	Bright	Oxyhaemoglobin Fe^{2+}	Behaves as water
Acute (3 h – 3 days)	Isointense	Dark	Deoxyhaemoglobin Fe^{2+}	Susceptibility effect
Subacute (3 days – 1 week)	Bright	Dark	Methaemoglobin Fe^{3+}	Intact red blood cells (RBC)
Subacute late (1 week – a few months)	Bright	Bright	Methaemoglobin Fe^{3+}	RBC lysis, liquid haemoglobin
Chronic (Months – years)	Dark	Dark	Ferritin/ haemosiderin Fe^{3+}	Crystalline storage form of iron

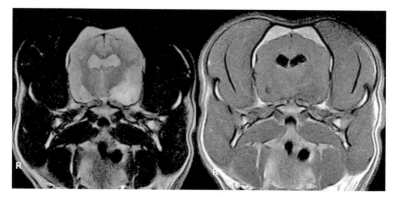

Figure 6.10 T2W high signal and T1W low signal appearances of a cerebral infarct.

accidents in dogs are usually cerebral, they may occur in the brainstem or cerebellum (Figure 6.11).

Trauma

The use of MRI in cases of acute trauma is severely limited by problems of urgent availability. Ideally, trauma cases require instant imaging and management. Nevertheless, MRI can be useful in demonstrating intracranial damage associated with head

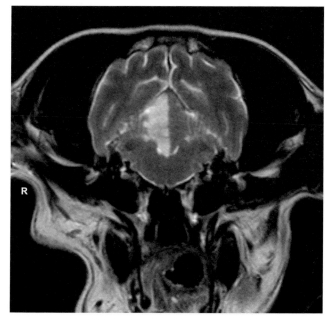

Figure 6.11 T2W transverse section through the brain showing right-sided cerebellar infarct. Note that the lesion stops abruptly at the midline.

injury, for example, and assessing the late effects of these injuries. In all cases radiography should be used to complement the MRI study since damage to the skull will be seen more clearly with the help of radiographs.

Inflammation

MRI is extremely sensitive to early changes in brain tissue, particularly white matter. Consequently, MRI is very effective in detecting the changes brought about by intracranial infection and inflammation. Administration of a gadolinium-based contrast agent can also demonstrate enhancement of the meninges indicating meningitis (Figure 6.12). Post-contrast sequences are also useful in distinguishing brain abscesses from cysts. An abscess will demonstrate peripheral enhancement around the edges of a cystic lesion (Figure 6.13). Simple cysts, not possessing a capsule, show no enhancement.

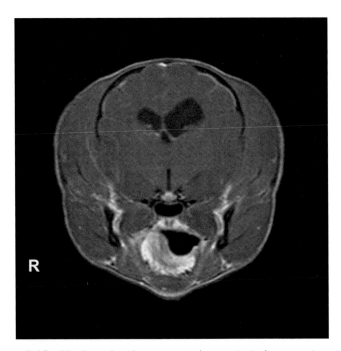

Figure 6.12 Meningeal enhancement demonstrated on post-contrast study of the brain.

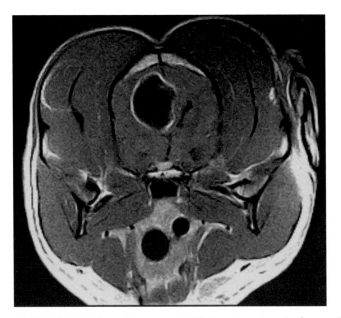

Figure 6.13 Typical ring enhancement (T1W post contrast) of a cerebral abcess.

In feline patients, feline infectious peritonitis (FIP) is also very nicely demonstrated; Figure 6.14 shows a post-contrast T1W dorsal section of a cat with intracranial FIP infection.

There are several non-infectious inflammatory diseases of the brain that regularly occur in dogs. Granulomatous meningoencephalitis (GME) has no breed predilection and occurs in both disseminated forms and a focal form. Necrotising meningoencephalitis (NME) was originally thought to be a breed-specific disease of the pug (Figure 6.15) but has now been recognised in several other small breeds. Necrotising encephalitis (NE) was first described in Yorkshire terriers but has recently been reported in the Boston terrier. Although there are similarities between these diseases they can be distinguished by biopsy and histopathological examination. The cause(s) of these encephalitides has not

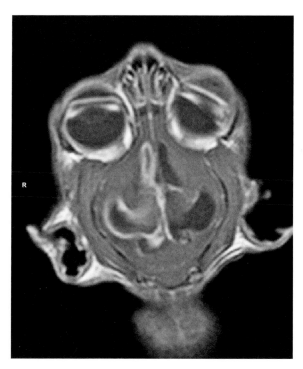

Figure 6.14 T1W dorsal section through the brain of a cat showing post-contrast enhancement typical of FIP.

USING MRI

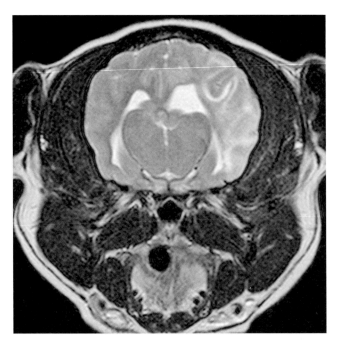

Figure 6.15 Transverse T2W section through the brain of a pug showing high signal in the left hemisphere typical of NME. Note that only slight midline shift is present.

been established but they are generally regarded as immunosuppressive processes. MRI reveals an appearance that is not pathognomonic but shows some characteristic lesion distribution. The lesions can be diffuse or focal; they are hyperintense on T2W due to the associated oedema and they are often, but not always, contrast-enhancing. Asymmetric ventricular dilatation is a consistent finding in NME.

Extracranial lesions

Extracranial neoplasia

Neoplastic lesions of the extracranial head and neck, including the orbits, are exquisitely demonstrated using MRI. The decision as to whether to proceed to surgery and subsequent surgical planning is greatly aided by MRI investigation. This can show the size, extent and spread of what, at first, can appear straightforward superficial lesions. Figure 6.16, for example, shows an extensive osteosarcoma that appears to be arising from the zygomatic arch. Note that the right orbit has been displaced and compressed by the mass. Figure 6.17 shows a similar mass, this time arising from the hard palate.

Where lesions can be shown to be superficial in nature with little or no infiltration or spread (Figure 6.18), surgery becomes a much more straightforward option.

Middle and inner ear

The degree of hyperintensity of abnormal contents of the middle ear cavity can give an indication of their nature. High signalling suggests that there is fluid exudate or a gel-like substance present. Less intensity indicates a thick or purulent exudate and low

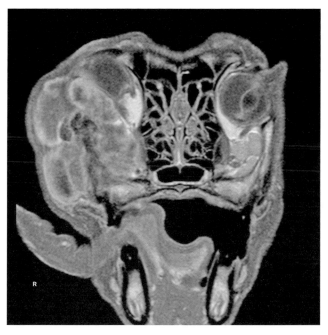

Figure 6.16 T2W transverse section showing an osteosarcoma arising from the zygomatic arch.

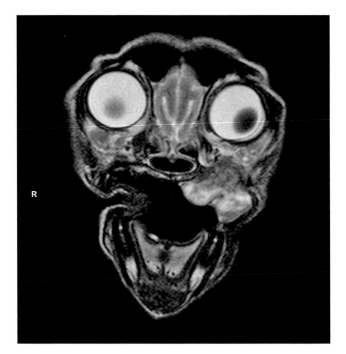

Figure 6.17 T2W transverse section showing a sarcoma of the hard palate.

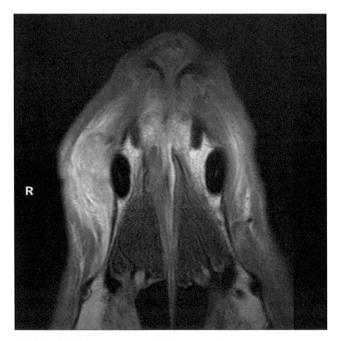

Figure 6.18 Soft tissue mass of the upper lip.

intensity suggests solid matter or tissue such as a polyp or other neoplasm (Figure 6.19).

The inner ear anatomy of dogs and cats is visualised very well on transverse images. Often the cochlea can be clearly distinguished because of its content of fluid endolymph. Again the degree of hyperintensity on T2 scans is significant, abnormally high signalling suggesting an inflammatory response.

Nasal abnormalities

Although radiography is used extensively in the investigation of nasal problems, the superior soft tissue differentiation of MRI means it is able to give much more information regarding the

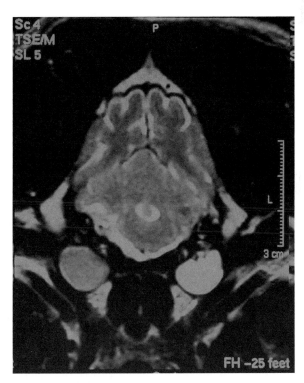

Figure 6.19 T2W transverse image showing abnormal signal from both tympanic bullae. The higher signal intensity on the left would suggest fluid.

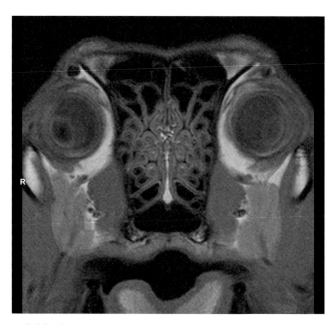

Figure 6.20 Transverse T1W section through the normal nasal turbinates.

nature of nasal lesions. The delicate anatomy of the nasal turbinates is particularly well demonstrated using MRI (Figure 6.20). Conditions such as chronic infection and nasal tumours can not only be identified, but MRI can demonstrate the size and extent of lesions as well as any growth across the bone into the cranium to involve the brain. *Aspergillus* infections are characterised by the visible erosion of the ethmoturbinates and the nasal septum. The presence of exudate or other pathology within the frontal sinuses is also very well visualised.

Spine

As with brain imaging, MRI has revolutionised the investigation and diagnosis of spinal disease. To be fair, veterinary surgeons did have at their disposal the ability to image the spinal cord indirectly by using myelography. This is an investigation still common in the veterinary field despite the fact that in human medicine it has been abandoned almost entirely for a number of years now. MRI is able to yield much more information, not least of all regarding the physical status of the spinal cord itself. The surrounding soft tissues, musculature and the inter-vertebral discs can all be assessed and, whilst MRI is not good for examining cortical bone, the technique is very sensitive to changes in bone marrow, a helpful feature when looking for spinal metastases.

MRI studies of the spine and spinal cord have revealed several features of anatomical interest. These are not abnormalities but are unexpected and the clinician should be aware of them to avoid mistaken diagnoses. The large size of the dorsal sub-arachnoid space in some large-breed dogs suggests that the spinal cord is abnormally small in diameter (Figure 6.21), but there is no functional disturbance. The dorsal longitudinal liga-ment forms part of the floor of the vertebral canal but can appear so prominent that it may be mistaken for an interverte-bral disc protrusion (Figure 6.22). MRI certainly demonstrates the great variation in the length of the spinal cord; in most dogs it ends at the level of the L6 vertebra but in some indi-viduals it is seen to extend as far as S2.

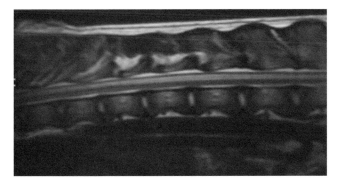

Figure 6.21 Sagittal T2W image of the caudal thoracic spine showing a capacious thecal sac giving the impression of a thinned spinal cord. This is a normal finding.

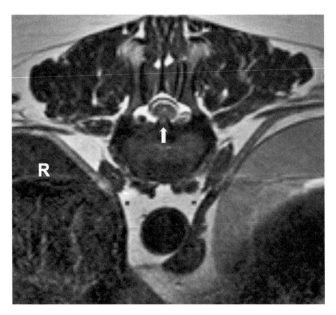

Figure 6.22 Transverse T2W section of the spine showing prominent dorsal longitudinal ligament (arrowed).

Intervertebral disc disease

Intervertebral disc disease (IVDD) is probably the major reason for carrying out an MR study of the spine. The ability to actually see an image of the spinal cord confers enormous advantages in the assessment of a disc protrusion/extrusion for both management and prognosis. Much has been written about the assessment of the clinical status based on the neurological signs demonstrated by the patient with IVDD. Pain perception in the limbs caudal to the lesion is certainly an important factor in assessing prognosis but inevitably it is very subjective – some dogs do not respond as readily as others and the clinician may be gentler than his/her colleagues. In the first place there has to be realisation that elicit-ing of spinal reflexes does not indicate pain perception and that a cerebral response is necessary. The duration of the 'loss of pain perception' is clearly another variable but is regarded as an accu-rate indication of prognosis, e.g. loss of deep pain sensation from the hindlimbs for a period of 4 h carries a poor prognosis and loss for 12h is hopeless. However, this generalisation has found frequent exceptions, 24 or even 48h of pain loss being followed by recovery.

It is interesting to interpret these criteria for prognosis in the light of MRI of the affected spinal cord. Scanning allows visualisation of intra- and extramedullary haemorrhage, intramedullary oedema and the exact degree of compression of the spinal cord by the extruded disc material. The actual appearance of the cord at the level of the disc protrusion may be more encouraging than the results of neurological examination, or it may be that what is seen allows an earlier certainty that the prognosis is hopeless.

Intervertebal disc protrusions and extrusions commonly occur in the cervical spine (Figure 6.23) and at the thoracolumbar

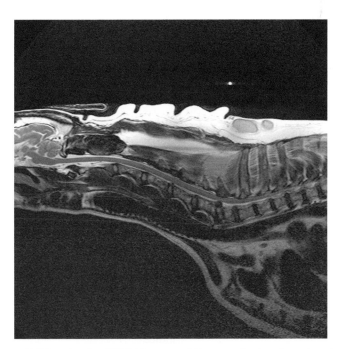

Figure 6.23 Sagittal T2W image of the cervical spine showing a protrusion of the intervertebral disc at C6/C7. There is also hypertrophy of the laminae causing dorsal compression of the spinal cord.

junction (Figure 6.24). MRI is very helpful in identifying these lesions, allowing an assessment of associated soft tissue damage and indicating appropriate surgical approaches, eg. left or right side for a hemilaminectomy (Figure 6.28). All three planes of orientation (Figures 6.25 and 6.26) should be used together with STIR sequences to provide the maximum amount of information. Multiple disc protrusions are not uncommon and emphasise the value of MRI in surgical planning (Figure 6.25). Ventral slot procedures for decompression of cervical spinal cord endanger the ventral venous sinuses so that it is useful to be able to see how much space is available for the slot.

The advantages of MRI for management of IVDD are simple but dramatic, for example radiography does not permit a transverse view of the spinal cord and although myelography may help it is not 100% reliable. The transverse oriented images of the cord in MRI give a clear visualisation of lateralisation of a disc protrusion (Figures 6.27–6.29) allowing a logical choice for the site of hemilaminectomy. MRI is superior to myelography, particularly in the assessment of lumbosacral disc disease (Figure 6.30) since the thecal sac often ends cranial to this level.

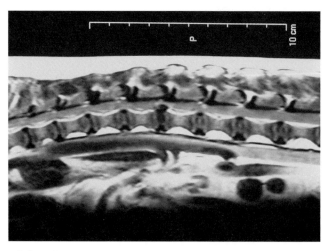

Figure 6.24 Sagittal T2W image of the thoracolumbar spine showing extrusion of the intervertebral disc at L1/L2.

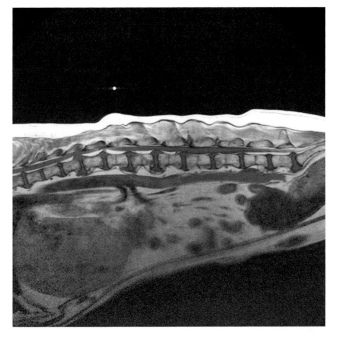

Figure 6.25 Sagittal T1W image of the thoracolumbar spine showing multiple intervertebral disc protrusions. Note the severe compression of the spinal cord at T12/T13.

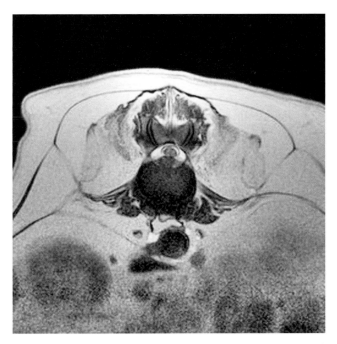

Figure 6.26 Transverse T1W slice of the thoracolumbar spine showing protrusion of the interverbral disc at T12/T13.

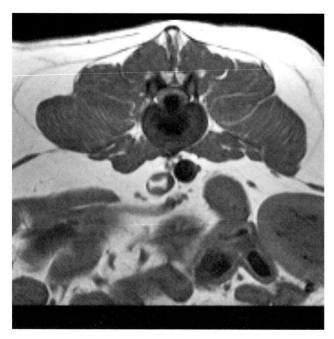

Figure 6.27 Central disc extrusion in the lumbar spine.

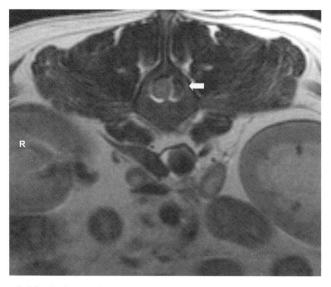

Figure 6.28 Left-sided disc extrusion in the lumbar spine (arrow).

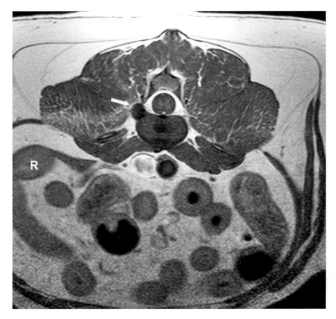

Figure 6.29 Far right-sided disc extrusion in the lumbar spine with migration of the disc material into the intervertebral foramen (arrow).

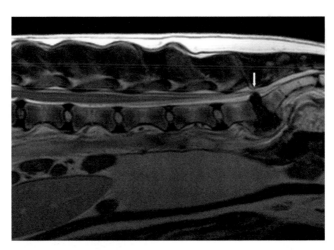

Figure 6.30 T2W sagittal image showing (arrowed) a lumbosacral disc protrusion.

Spinal neoplasia

Severe and progressive disturbance of spinal cord function is likely to be due to neoplasia within the vertebral canal. The relatively small cross-sectional area of the spinal cord (1.0–$1.5\,cm^2$ in a medium-sized dog) means that a tumour does not have to be very large to have a disastrous effect on the spinal cord. An intramedullary neoplasm (Figure 6.31) inevitably comes with a very poor prognosis but extramedullary tumours can often be excised successfully.

MRI of spinal neoplasia allows a precise assessment of the extent of the tumour and often the likely identity. Meningiomas (Figure 6.32) have frequent incidence in both dogs and cats; they are hyperintense on T2W and enhance brightly with gadolinium. They usually extend along the canal and are often soft and friable, making complete removal difficult. Nerve root tumours (Figure 6.33) are not uncommon and are usually identified by the extension of neoplastic tissue through an intervertebral foramen. Gliomas, lymphoid tumours and metastases are all seen and the clinical signs are related to the size, location and speed of pro-

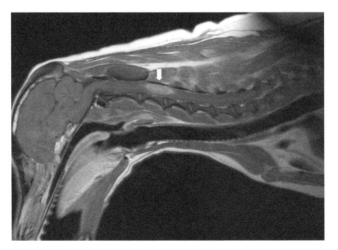

Figure 6.31 Post-contrast study demonstrating intramedullary neoplasia (arrow).

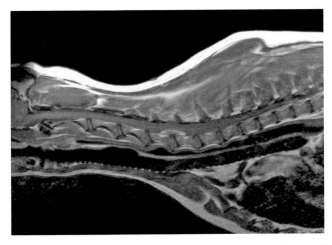

Figure 6.32 Post-contrast study demonstrating a meningioma adjacent to the C5–6 disc space.

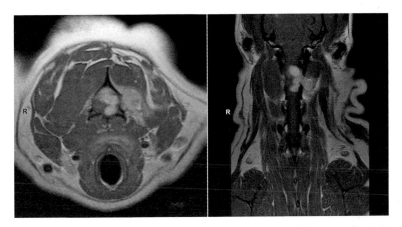

Figure 6.33 T1W post-contrast transverse and dorsal images of a left-sided cervical nerve root tumour.

gression. STIR sequences are particularly useful for locating spinal cord tumours and the dorsal orientation is usually essential.

Tumours of the vertebrae and paraspinal tissues are also seen (Figure 6.34) and may well cause localised compression of the spinal cord. Although radiography will usually be necessary to

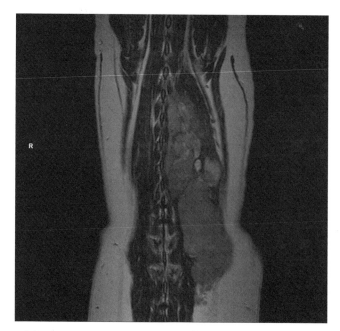

Figure 6.34 T2W dorsal section demonstrating a very large left-sided paraspinal mass.

visualise a bone tumour, MRI is helpful in assessing the involvement of the spinal cord (Figure 6.35).

Vascular lesions

The spinal cord has an extensive anastomosing blood supply. Nevertheless there are frequent instances in which the blood vessels to one or more segments of cord become damaged or occluded. The resulting ischaemia causes rapid dysfunction, e.g. limb paresis, proprioceptive deficits, etc. The commonest example of this situation is a fibrocartilaginous embolism (FCE) (Figure 6.36), visualised by MRI as a small localised region of hyperintensity on T2W, representing the resulting intramedullary oedema. Traumatic damage to blood vessels within the vertebral canal (e.g. the vertebral venous sinuses) may result in extramedullary

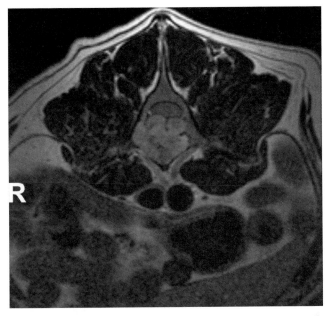

Figure 6.35 Transverse T2W section demonstrating a vertebral body tumour compressing the spinal cord.

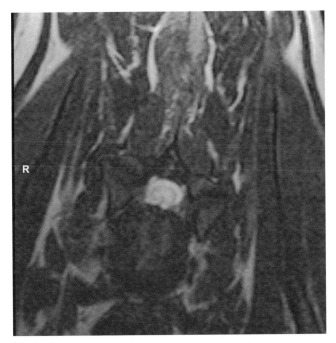

Figure 6.36 Transverse T2W section demonstrating fibrocartilaginous embolism.

haemorrhage, seen on MRI T2W scans as an elongated region of hyperintensity.

Myelomalacia is a progressive pathological condition in which the spinal cord becomes so severely damaged through ischaemia that it appears liquefied. The MRI findings in myelomalacia are of an intramedullary region of hyperintensity on both T1W and T2W. Spinal haemorrhage often shows the characteristic susceptibility artefact due the breakdown of blood products (Figure 6.37).

Trauma

Spinal injuries in dogs are fairly common and are usually the result of road traffic accidents. Whereas radiography is the imaging technique of choice for assessing damage to vertebrae, MRI scanning is invaluable for visualising and assessing damage to the spinal cord (Figure 6.38). Fractures/dislocations of the vertebrae are easily seen with the use of X-rays but MRI is needed to identify cord transection, haemorrhage and oedema (Figure 6.39). In most circumstances when scanning is within 24–48 h, the characteristic change in signalling to focal or diffuse hyperintensity on T2W images suggests cord injury. It is true that cord injury can occur without vertebral damage and MRI will then localise the problem when radiography cannot.

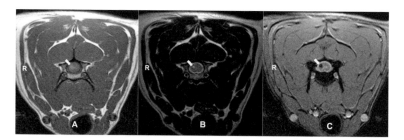

Figure 6.37 Three transverse sections taken at the same anatomical level of the cervical spine showing the appearances of spinal cord bleed (arrows) on (A) T1W SE, (B) T2W TSE and (C) T2*W GE, showing characteristic susceptibility artefact from haemorrhage.

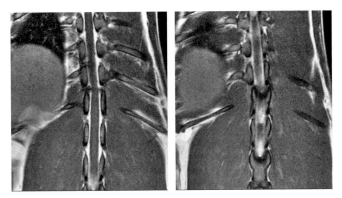

Figure 6.38 Dorsal T1W sections of the thoracolumbar spine at the level of a spinal fracture.

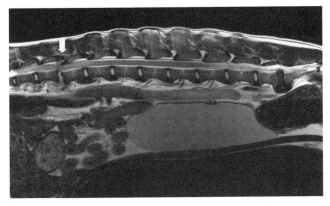

Figure 6.39 T2W sagittal section of the same spinal fracture shown in Figure 6.38. Note spinal cord oedema adjacent to T13 vertebral body.

Infection

Infection invariably triggers a local reaction ranging from lymphoedema to abscess formation. MRI is very sensitive to these changes and can demonstrate infective processes exquisitely. Probably the most common infection found in the spinal region is that associated with discospondylitis (Figure 6.40). Commonly, a degenerative disc will become infected often leading to damage of the adjacent end plates with changes spreading to the nearby bone

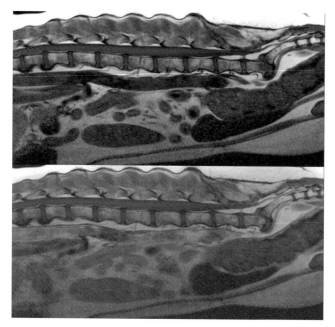

Figure 6.40 T1W sagittal sections before (top) and after the administration of intravenous contrast. The post-contrast image (bottom) shows enhancement in the caudal region of the L7 vertebra due to discospondylitis.

marrow. Administration of intravenous contrast agent will result in enhancement where the process is still active due to the patent vascularity of the tissues.

Degenerative disease

Degenerative disease is certainly the most common cause of spinal problems in small animals. Degenerative disc disease is well demonstrated using MRI (Figures 6.41 and 6.42). On T2W a normal healthy disc has a hyperintense centre (the nucleus pulposus) and the change to hypointensity as the disc dehydrates indicates degeneration. Whilst not strictly degenerative pathology, other processes such as ligament and facet joint hypertrophy (Figure 6.43) are equally well demonstrated.

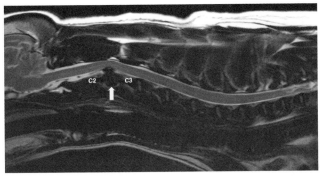

Figure 6.41 T2W sagital section showing obvious disc prolapse but note also the loss of signal from the C2–3 disc indicating dehydration.

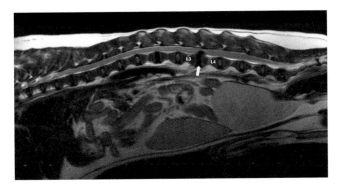

Figure 6.42 Lumbar disc degeneration with associated disc prolapse at L3–4.

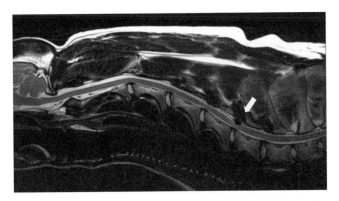

Figure 6.43 Sagittal T2W image showing cord compression and associated cord oedema at the level of C5–6. In this instance compression is dorsal and the disc appears normal.

Many degenerative conditions of the central nervous system have been described and the incidence in dogs is quite high. Unfortunately, with a few exceptions, MRI has limited use as a diagnostic tool for these diseases. Chronic degenerative radiculo-myelopathy (CDRM) occurs most commonly in German Shepherd Dogs of 7–10 years of age. It has a characteristic clinical presentation, progressive course and post-mortem appearance. However, evidence of CDRM is rarely visible by MRI scanning; it becomes rather a diagnosis by elimination once it is clear that evidence of intervertebral disc disease is not present.

The situation is a little better with degenerative brain disease in that some conditions do have characteristic MRI findings. Certainly cerebellar (Figure 6.44) and cerebrocortical atrophy can be identified. L-2-hydroxyglutaric aciduria (L-2-HGA) is an example of a degenerative disease of the brain with a characteristic appearance on MRI. It is an inherited disorder of neuron metabolism

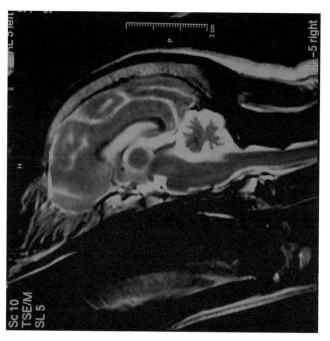

Figure 6.44 Cerebellar atrophy.

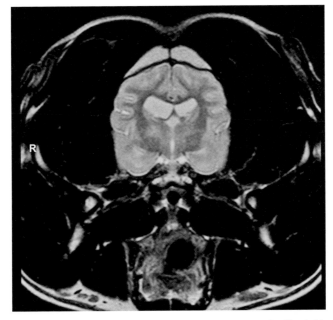

Figure 6.45 Transverse T2W study of the brain in a Staffordshire bull terrier showing characteristic MRI appearances of L-2-HGA.

occurring in the Staffordshire bull terrier. The clinical signs are variable but seizures, dementia, muscle tremors and ataxia are commonly reported. The findings on MRI are within the grey matter, mainly of the cerebrum and cerebellum and are seen as bilaterally symmetrical, multifocal areas of moderate hyperintensity on T2W scans (Figure 6.45).

Congenital abnormalities

When young animals present with neurological abnormalities, congenital anomalies must be high on the list of possible causes. MRI is an excellent method of assessing the brain and CSF pathway system for a range of abnormalities from hydrocephalus, which can be glaringly obvious (Figure 6.46), to structural brain

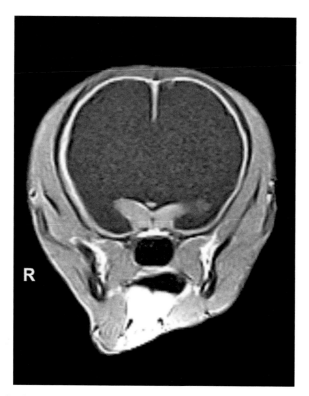

Figure 6.46 Gross hydrocephalus.

anomalies such as that demonstrated in Figure 6.47 where the corpus callosum is absent.

Whilst many skeletal congenital abnormalities are plainly visible on radiographs, MRI has the added advantage of being able to demonstrate associated soft tissue involvement such as nerve root entrapment, spinal cord compression and abnormalities of the thecal sac and spinal cord itself. Kyphosis and scoliosis occur regularly in certain breeds; MRI provides the opportunity to assess the effect on the spinal cord, helping to determine management and prognosis (Figure 6.48).

Figure 6.49 shows a dorsal oblique view along the sacrum of a dog with a transitional vertebra. The right side shows a normal sacro-iliac joint whilst on the left there is a transverse process

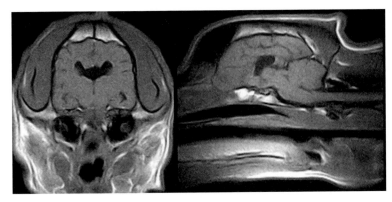

Figure 6.47 T1W Sagittal and transverse images in a young dog with no apparent corpus callosum.

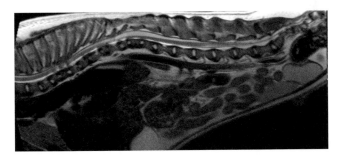

Figure 6.48 T2W sagittal section in a bulldog with radiographically demonstrated congenital spinal anomalies.

more in keeping with a lumbar vertebra. Figure 6.50 shows the same anomaly in transverse section.

It could be argued that more complex conditions such as the Chiari-like malformation, which occurs commonly in Cavalier King Charles spaniels, can only be assessed fully using MRI. All affected individuals possess a malformation of the foramen magnum; it is larger than normal and usually is extended dorsally. The consequence of this abnormality is herniation of the caudal region of the cerebellar vermis. This is very clearly seen on scans in the sagittal plane (Figure 6.51). The occlusion of the foramen magnum results in interruption of the flow of CSF into the cisterna magna

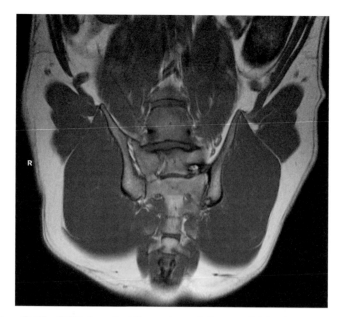

Figure 6.49 T1W dorsal oblique view of the caudal lumbar spine and sacrum showing a transitional vertebra. On the left side there is a transverse process consistent with a lumbar vertebra whilst on the right there is a clear sacro-iliac joint.

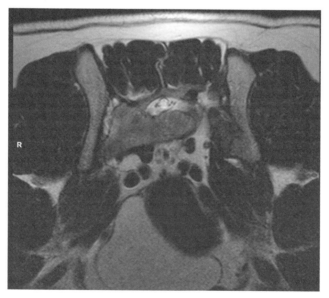

Figure 6.50 Transverse view of the anomaly shown in Figure 6.49.

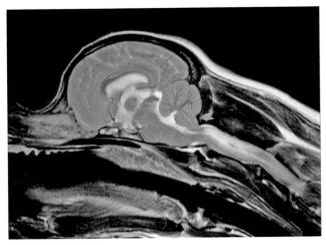

Figure 6.51 Sagittal T2W section through the cranio-cervical region of a Cavalier King Charles spaniel showing cerebellar herniation (chevron).

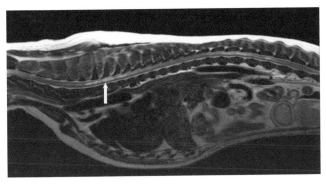

Figure 6.52 Characteristic T2W high signal cavitation of the spinal cord indicating syrinx formation.

and redirection of the CSF into the central canal. MRI scans of affected dogs may show dilated ventricles and the presence of a syrinx (syringohydromyelia) within the spinal cord (Figure 6.52).

Hydrocephalus is a dilatation of the ventricular system of the brain; it arises either as an acquired condition or it may be congenital in origin. The size of the lateral ventricles in an affected dog may be so large that only a thin layer of brain parenchyma surrounds the fluid-filled cavities (Figure 6.53). The CSF is hypointense on T1W and hyperintense on T2W scans.

Arachnoid cysts are often seen on MR images of the spine; they do not necessarily result in clinical signs.

Congenital abnormalities of the vertebrae are demonstrated better by radiography than by MRI. However, MRI provides visualisation of the spinal cord and an assessment, together with the clinical signs, of the likely functional disturbance and prognosis. The advantages of being able to assess the effects of bony abnormality on the soft tissues again emphasise the way in which radiography complements MRI.

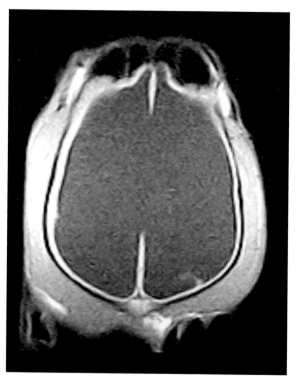

Figure 6.53 Dorsal T1W image of severe hydrocephalus. The cerebral parenchyma is almost non-existent.

Musculoskeletal system

The use of MRI is becoming increasingly common as a non-invasive and effective way of examining joints. In particular, the shoulder (Figure 6.54), elbow (Figure 6.55) and stifle (Figure 6.56) are often examined in cases of trauma or suspected degenerative disease; ligament ruptures, meniscal tears, tendonitis etc. are all well demonstrated. Of course it could be argued that arthroscopy, where available, can provide this information whilst facilitating therapeutic intervention at the same time. MRI, however, is often more widely available these days and is non-invasive.

MRI comes into its own when visualising structures outside the joint capsule and in the adjacent bones (Figure 6.57) or the investigation of soft tissues of the limbs. MRI is essential in the assessment of the nature and extent of soft tissue masses (Figure 6.58) where surgical intervention is being considered.

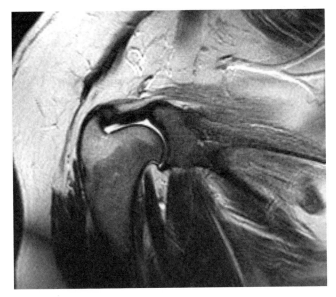

Figure 6.54   T2*W GE oblique section of the shoulder.

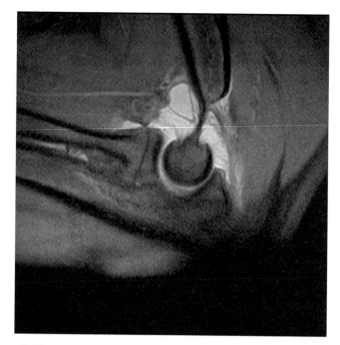

Figure 6.55 PDW sagittal section of the elbow. The use of a fat saturation pulse clearly demontrates the high signal fluid within the joint capsule.

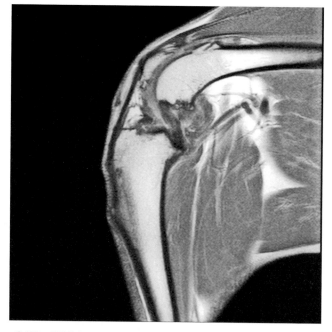

Figure 6.56 T1W image of the stifle joint.

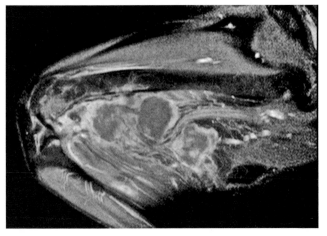

Figure 6.57 Post-contrast study of the hindlimb. T1W with fat saturation shows extensive tumour behind the stifle joint with involvement of the distal femur.

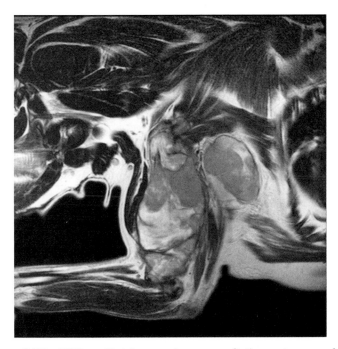

Figure 6.58 T2W sagittal image shows a soft tissue tumour of the proximal forelimb with extension into the chest wall ruling out forelimb amputation.

Thorax, abdomen and pelvis

This is an area of MRI study that is still very much in its infancy, particularly in the field of veterinary medicine. Ultrasound is often more widely available, cheaper and, in the hands of a competent practitioner, more effective than MRI. That is not to say that MRI does not have a place in the study of these regions. In the pelvis, where physiological movement is not so much of an issue, very good results are obtainable with even basic equipment (Figure 6.59). Sophisticated high field MR systems with respiratory gating and motion reduction software can produce very acceptable abdominal images (Figure 6.60). Even in the thorax where MRI is sometimes regarded as being of little value, useful information can often be obtained, for example when investigating mediastinal masses (Figure 6.61).

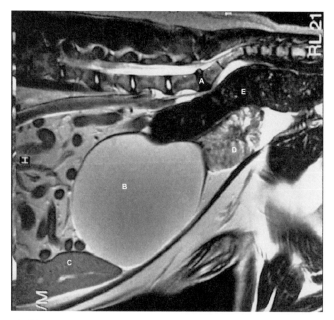

Figure 6.59 Low field T2W image of the pelvis showing: (A) lumbosacral disc disease, (B) urinary bladder, (C) caudal spleen, (D) prostate gland and (E) rectum.

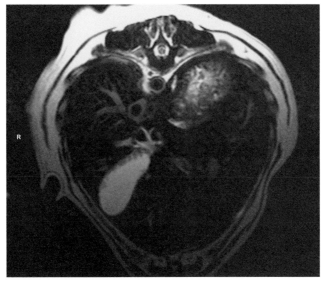

Figure 6.60 Transverse T2W section through the liver obtained using respiratory gating shows multiple stones within the gall bladder.

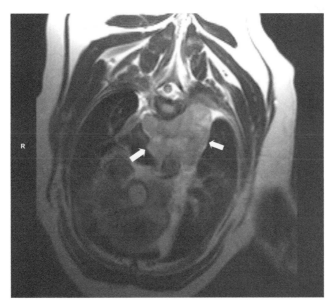

Figure 6.61 Transverse T2W section through the chest obtained using respiratory gating. A mediastinal mass adjacent to the spine is clearly visible (arrowed).

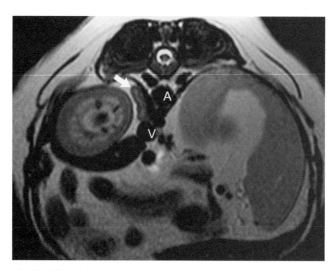

Figure 6.62   The right adrenal gland (arrow) shown on a respiratory gated transverse T2W study of the abdomen. The gland lies in close approximation to the aorta (A) and the caudal vena cava (V).

The urogenital organs can be examined usefully with MRI, especially well circumscribed, easily identifiable structures such as the ovaries and prostate. In most circumstances the examination will determine the presence or absence of neoplasia and the extent of the lesion as a prerequisite for surgery. The location of the adrenal glands, either side of the aorta and close to the renal arteries, make them relatively easy to identify so that they can be examined with MRI for pathological changes (Figure 6.62). This is particularly appropriate if the animal has been anaesthetised to examine the pituitary in the case of Cushing's disease, for example.

As experience grows this area of imaging will continue to reap benefits and users should not be afraid to 'experiment' appropriately in these areas.

Foreign bodies

MRI has a place in the location and identification of foreign bodies that are not radiopaque. Wooden splinters etc. can often be visualised indirectly due to their absence of signal (signal void) and may be found because of an inflammatory reaction or accumulation of fluid in association with the foreign body (Figure 6.63). Tracts from foreign bodies to the periphery may be identified and then 'followed' by scanning to allow the determination of anatomical landmarks to facilitate surgical removal (Figure 6.64). Metallic foreign bodies are sometimes incidental findings, especially in the gastrointestinal tract; they are not seen as clearly identifiable shapes but rather as distortions of the image. Ferrous metals may move and become heated; scanning should be stopped immediately to avoid damage to the adjacent tissues. Patients may be scanned at a later date once radiography has shown that foreign bodies have been passed.

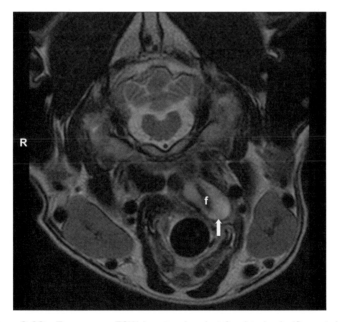

Figure 6.63 Transverse T2W image showing foreign body (f) contained within a fluid-filled abcess (arrow). In this case there was no definite history of foreign body.

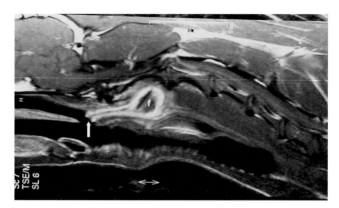

Figure 6.64 Pharyngeal stick injury. In this case the entry wound was clearly visible (arrow) but the foreign body (f) was found some distance away adjacent to the body of C2.

Anatomy Atlas for MRI Interpretation

This section illustrates a selection of anatomical terms. It is not an exhaustive list but does draw attention to the organs and structures that are the most important for recognising abnormality on MR images. The English versions of the terms have been used but wherever possible the terms are the equivalent of those listed in *Nomina Anatomica Veterinaria.*

Anatomical illustrations have been chosen for their frequent usage in veterinary clinical applications of MRI. Some regions have not been included (e.g. extremities and some joints) because they are infrequent subjects for MRI and are more suitably studied by computed tomography. To avoid unnecessary repetition only a small number of slices have been illustrated in each orientation and, although structures may appear on several slices, they are not always labelled.

The abbreviations have been chosen to provide a logical representation of the anatomical terms and in most cases the name abbreviated will be obvious.

MRI scans of the brain – abbreviations

basa	basilar artery	mo	medulla oblongata
caq	cerebral (mesence-phalic) aqueduct	nc	nasal cavity
		nph	nasopharynx
cb	cerebellum	ol	occipital lobe
cbr	cerebrum	olf	olfactory lobe
cc	central canal	opc	optic chiasma
cca	corpus callosum	opn	optic nerve
crp	cribriform plate	pb	parietal bone
cw	circle of Willis	pfl	piriform lobe
dnme	dorsal nasal meatus	pit	pituitary gland (hypophysis)
el	endoturbinate I		
ell	endoturbinate II	pl	parietal lobe
elll	endoturbinate III	po	pons
extme	external meatus	rl	rostral lobe (of cerebellum)
fb	frontal bone		
fl	frontal lobe	sp	soft palate
fs	frontal sinus	tb	tympanic bulla
fx	falx cerebri	tent	tentorium cerebelli
glp	globus pallidus	tg	tongue
gtcv	great cerebral vein	th	thalamus
hip	hippocampus	tl	temporal lobe
ica	internal carotid artery	tm	temporalis muscle
		vcn	vestibulocochlear nerve
ie	inner ear		
intad	interthalamic adhesion	vncon	ventral nasal concha
latv	lateral ventricle	vnme	ventral nasal meatus
linga	lingual artery		
mb	midbrain	III	third ventricle
me	middle ear	IV	fourth ventricle

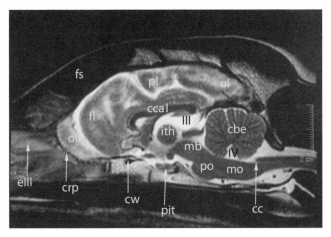

SAG Brain

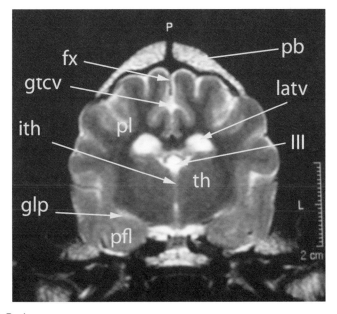

TRA Brain

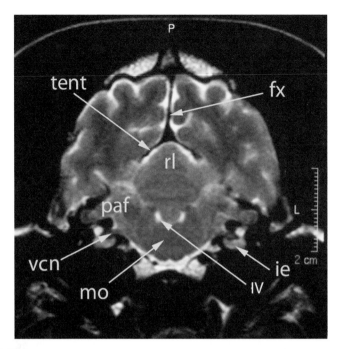

TRA Brain

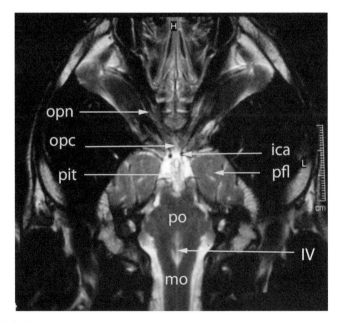

DOR Brain

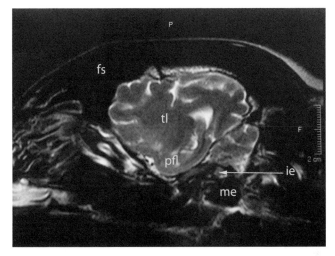

SAG Brain

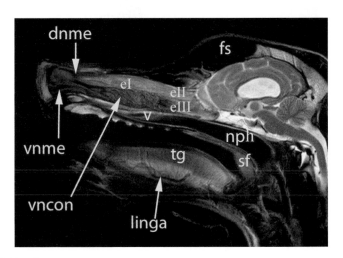

SAG Head

MRI scans of the spine – abbreviations

af	anulus fibrosus	ivj	intervertebral joint
am	arachnoid mater	np	nucleus pulposus
ca	coeliac artery	oe	oesophagus
ceq	cauda equina	r	rectum
cm	cisterna magna	s	spleen
cma	cranial mesenteric	sa	sacrum
	artery	sc	spinal cord
d	dens	si	small intestine
da	dorsal aorta	sij	sacroiliac joint
dm	dura mater	suba	subarachnoid space
epi	epidural space	tra	trachea
for	intervertebral foramen	ub	urinary bladder
il	ilium	vb	vertebral body

Vertebrae are numbered as follows C7, T13, L1, S2 etc.

Intervertebral discs are numbered according to the adjacent vertebrae eg. L7/S1.

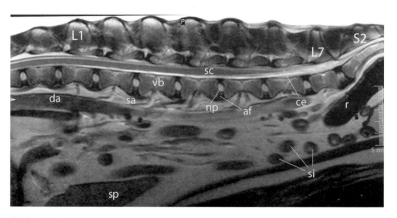

SAG Lumbosacral spine

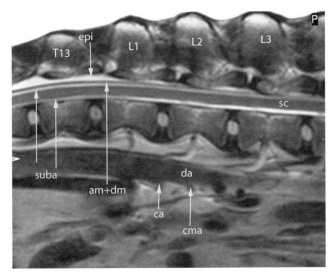

SAG Thoracolumbar junction

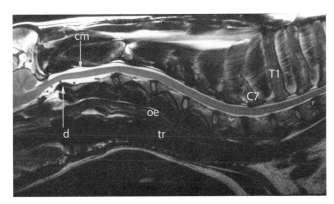

SAG Cervical spine

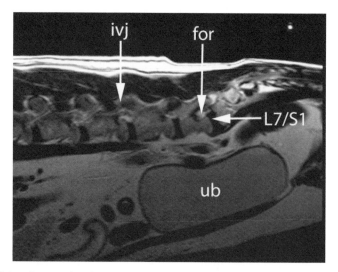

SAG Lumbosacral spine

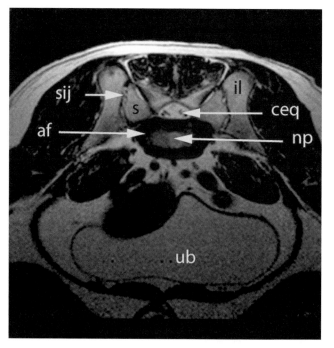

TRA Lumbosacral junction

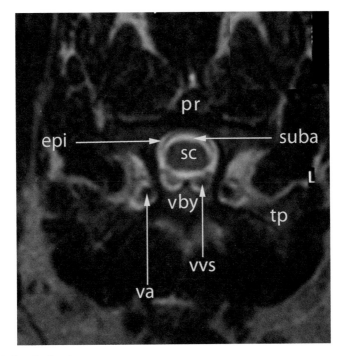

TRA Cervical spine

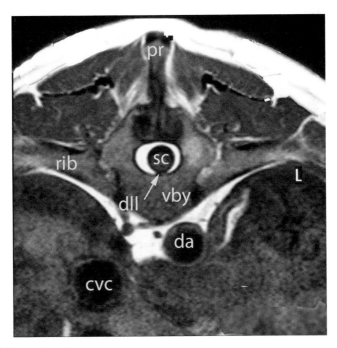

TRA Thoracic spine

MRI scans of the abdomen – abbreviations

ac	ascending colon	lra	left renal artery
by	body of stomach	pa	pancreas
ca	coeliac artery	portv	hepatic portal vein
cma	cranial mesenteric artery	pt	prostate gland
		py	pyloric part of stomach
cmv	cranial mesenteric vein	ql	quadrate lobe (of liver)
col	colon	r	rectum
cvc	caudal vena cava	rlatl	right lateral lobe (liver)
da	dorsal aorta	rmel	right medial lobe (liver)
dc	descending colon	rra	right renal artery
du	duodenum	sc	spinal cord
fu	fundic part of stomach	si	small intestine
gb	gall bladder	sp	spleen
k	kidney	st	stomach
lag	left adrenal gland	tc	transverse colon
lmel	left medial lobe (liver)	ub	urinary bladder

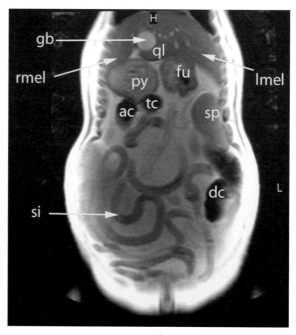

DOR Abdomen

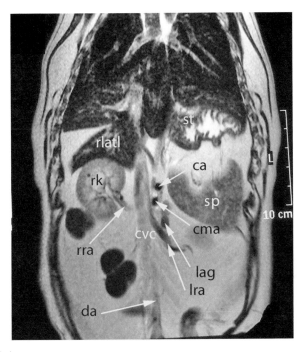

DOR Abdomen

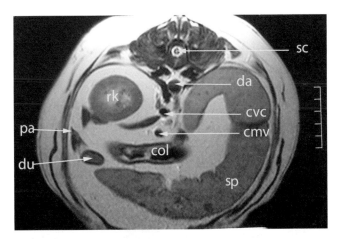

TRA Abdomen (level of right kidney)

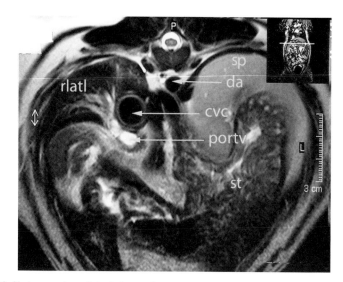

TRA Abdomen (cranial abdomen)

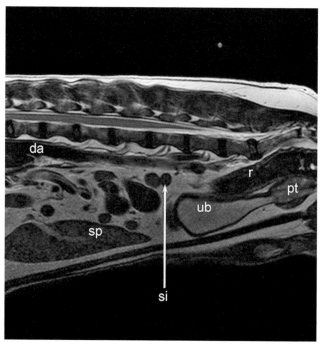

SAG Pelvis

MRI scans of joints – abbreviations

artcar	articular cartilage	longdem	long digital extensor muscle
bicepst	biceps tendon		
bifem	biceps femoris muscle	mcoll	medial collateral ligament
cacrl	caudal cruciate ligament	mfab	medial fabella
		mfeco	medial femoral condyle
cbram	cleidobrachialis muscle	pal	patellar ligament
crcrl	cranial cruciate ligament	pat	patella
		popa	popliteal artery
fat	infrapatellar fat pad	popm	popliteus muscle
		popv	popliteal vein
fe	femur	scapsp	scapular spine
gastrocm	gastrocnemius muscle	scaptub	scapular tuberosity
gttub	greater tuberosity	supm	supraspinatus muscle
hhead	humeral head		
lcoll	lateral collateral ligament	sycav	synovial cavity
		tib	tibia
lfab	lateral fabella	tibtb	tibial tuberosity
lfeco	lateral femoral condyle	tribram	triceps brachii muscle
lgastroc	lateral gastrocnemius muscle		

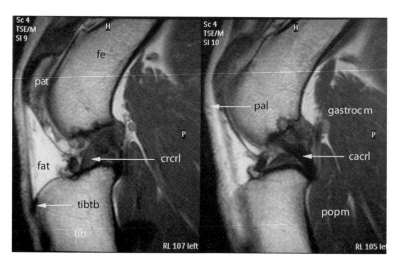

MED Stifle

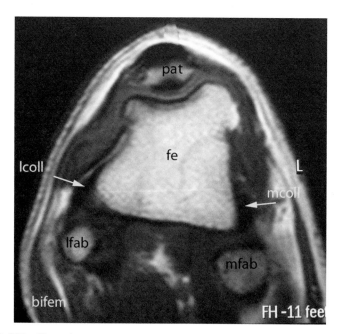

TRA Stifle (femur)

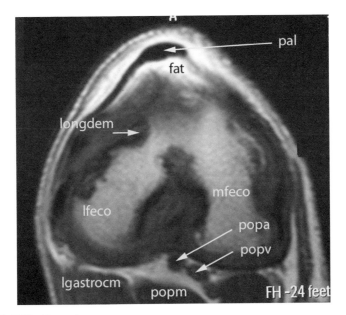

TRA Stifle (femur)

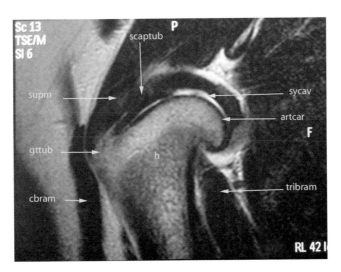

MED Shoulder

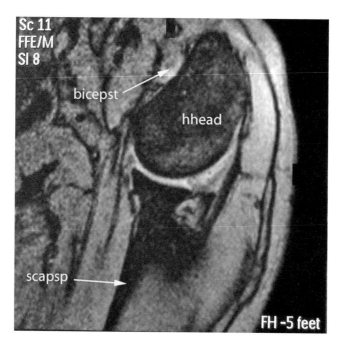

MED Shoulder

Further Reading

Adams, W.H., Daniel, G.B., Pardo, A.D. and Selcer, R.R. (1995) Magnetic resonance imaging of the caudal lumbar and lumbosacral spine in 13 dogs (1990–1993). *Veterinary Radiology and Ultrasound*, **36**, 1.

Assheuer, J. and Sager, M. (1997) *MRI and CT Atlas of the Dog*. Blackwell Publishing Ltd., Oxford.

Chambers, J.N., Selcer, R.A., Sullivan S.A. *et al.* (1997) Diagnosis of lateralized lumbosacral disk herniation with magnetic resonance imaging. *Journal of the American Animal Hospital Association*, **33** (4), 296–9.

Coates, J.R. (2000) Intervertebral disc disease. *Veterinary Clinics of North America (Small Animal Practice)*, **30** (1), 77–110.

deHaan, J.J., Shelton, S.B. and Ackerman, N. (1993) Magnetic resonance imaging in the diagnosis of degenerative lumbosacral stenosis in four dogs. *Veterinary Surgery*, **22** (1), 1–4.

Dobromylsky, M.J., Dennis, R., Ladlow, J.F. *et al.* (2007) The use of magnetic resonance imaging in the management of pharyngeal penetration injuries in dogs. *Journal of Small Animal Practice* (On line early article) Sep 2007.

Farrow, C.S. and Tryon, K. (2000) Fathoming the mysteries of magnetic resonance imaging. *Journal of the American Animal Hospital Association*, **36** (3), 192–8.

Feeney, D.A., Fletcher, T.F and Hardy R.M. (1991) *Atlas of Correlative Imaging Anatomy of the Normal Dog*. WB Saunders, Philadelphia.

Francisco, J., Llabres-Diaz, V.M.B. and Dennis, R. (2003) Magnetic resonance imaging of the presumed normal canine adrenal glands. *Veterinary Radiology and Ultrasound*, **44** (1), 5–19.

Gandini, G., Cizinauskas, S., Lang, J. *et al.* (2003) Fibrocartilagenous embolism in 75 dogs: clinical findings and factors influencing the recovery rate. *Journal of Small Animal Practice*, **44** (2), 76–80.

Hudson, L.C., Cauzinille, L., Kornegay, J.N. *et al.* (1995) Magnetic resonance imaging of the normal feline brain. *Veterinary Radiology and Ultrasound*, **36** (4), 267–75.

Kippenes, H., Gavin, P.R., Bagley, R.S. *et al.* (1999) Magnetic resonance imaging features of tumours of the spine and spinal cord. *Veterinary Radiology and Ultrasound*, **40** (6), 627–33.

Kraft, S.L., Gavin, P.R., Wendling, L.R. *et al.* (1989) Canine brain anatomy on magnetic resonance images. *Veterinary Radiology* **30** (4), 147–58.

Lipsitz, D., Levitski, R.E., Chauvet, A.E. *et al.* (2001) Magnetic resonance imaging features of cervical stenotic myelopathy in 21 dogs. *Veterinary Radiology and Ultrasound*, **42** (1), 20–7.

Parker, A.J., Adams, W.M. and Zachary, J.F. (1983) Spinal arachnoid cysts in the dog. *Journal of the American Animal Hospital Association*, **19**, 1001–8.

Petite, A.F.B. and Dennis, R. (2006) Comparison of radiography and magnetic resonance imaging for evaluating the extent of nasal neoplasia in dogs. *Journal of Small Animal Practice*, **47** (9), 529–36.

Platt, S.R. and Garosi, L. (2003) Canine cerebrovascular disease: do dogs have strokes. *Journal of the American Animal Hospital Association*, **39** (4), 337–42.

Runge, V.M. (2002) *Clinical MRI*. WB Saunders Co., Philadelphia.

Shores, A. (1993) Magnetic resonance imaging. *Veterinary Clinics of North America (Small Animal Practice)*, **23** (2), 437–59.

Simpson, S.T. (1992) Intervertebral disc disease. *Veterinary Clinics of North America (Small Animal Practice)*, **22**, 889–97.

Sukhiani, H.R., Parent, J.M., Atilola, M.A. *et al.* (1996) Intervertebral disc disease in dogs with signs of back pain alone: 25 cases (1986–1993). *Journal of the Amercan Veterinary Medical Association*, **209**, 1275–9.

Thomas, W.B., Wheeler, S.J., Kramer, R. *et al.* (1996) Magnetic resonance imaging features of primary brain tumours in dogs. *Veterinary Radiology and Ultrasound*, **37** (1), 20–27.

Thomson, C.E., Kornegay, J.N., Burns, R.A. *et al.* (1993) Magnetic resonance imaging – a general overview of principles and examples in veterinary neurodiagnostics. *Veterinary Radiology and Ultrasound*, **34** (1), 2–17.

Westbrook, C. and Kaut, C. (1993) *MRI in Practice*. Blackwell Publishing, Oxford.

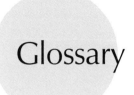

Glossary

Aliasing	Artefact caused when anatomy which is larger than the field of view in the phase direction is 'folded over' and misrepresented in the image. Also known as 'phase wrap' or 'foldover'.
Atomic number	The number of protons in the nucleus of an atom.
B_0	Denotes the main magnetic field as opposed to secondary fields created by gradient coils.
Chemical shift	An artefact occuring in the frequency direction as a result of the different precessional frequency of hydrogen in fat and water.
Cryogens	The liquid gases (invariably helium but nitrogen was also used in older systems) used to cool the windings of superconducting magnets.
CSF	Cerebrospinal fluid.
Decay	Reduction of the transverse component of the net magnetisation vector (NMV).
Dephasing	Loss of synchronisation of the precessional paths of nuclei in the transverse plane.
Echo train length	ETL. The number of phase encoding steps aquired per TR in fast spin echo imaging. Also known as 'turbo factor'.

Excitation	An increase in net magnetisation arising from energy imparted by an RF pulse.
Faraday cage	The lining of the scanning room, designed to keep extraneous radiofrequency signals from being detected by the receiver coil.
Fast spin echo	FSE. A fast imaging sequence also referred to by some manufacturers as turbo spin echo (TSE).
Fat saturation	A method of eliminating signal from fat by applying a saturation pulse tuned to the precessional frequency of hydrogen in fat.
Field of view	FOV. The area of anatomy included in an image.
Flip angle	The angle through which the net magnetisation vector (NMV) passes as a result of the applied RF pulse. Usually 90 or 180° but other flip angles are used in gradient echo sequences.
Flow artefact	Misrepresentation of MR signals in the image caused by movement of nuclei during the image acquisition.
Flow phenomena	A blanket term for the image appearances resulting from flowing nuclei, usually in blood or CSF.
Fluid attenuated inversion recovery	FLAIR. A sequence used in brain and spinal imaging to eliminate signal from water (CSF).
Fourier transform	A mathematical process whereby the data acquired in K space is converted to greyscale values needed to create an image.
Free induction decay	FID. The loss of signal detected by the receiver coil following termination of the applied RF pulse.
Fringe fields	Unwanted and potentially hazardous magnetic fields occuring outside the confines of the MR scanner.
Gauss	A unit of measurement of magnetic field. 10 000 Gauss = 1 Tesla.

Ghosting	Another name for movement artefact.
Gradient echo	An echo resulting from the application of a gradient refocusing.
Gyromagnetic ratio	A mathematical constant which describes an element's ability to resonate, usually expressed as the precessional frequency of the element at 1 T.
Homogeneity	The uniformity of magnetic field.
Image weighting	The predominance within an image of a particular contrast type: T1, T2 or PD.
Inhomogeneities	Variations in uniformity of the magnetic field.
Isocentre	The centre of the MR scanner in all planes of orientation.
K space	Prior to conversion into an image, signals received are stored in 'K space'.
Larmor equation	The mathematical formula used to determine the precessional frequency of an element at a given field strength.
Magneto-optical disc	MOD. A digital storage medium.
Net magnetisation vector	NMV. The total strength and direction of all magnetic vectors in a sample.
Peak amplitude	The maximum steepness achievable by gradient coils.
PD	*Protein density*
Phase	The position of the hydrogen proton on its precessional path at any moment in time.
Phase encoding	The spatial localisation of a nucleus according to its phase at the time of signal readout.
Pixel	Two-dimensional picture element affecting area resolution.
Precession	The movement of spinning magnetic moments around B_0.
Presaturation	The use of a saturation pulse to eliminate signals from moving tissue.

Pulse sequence	The sequence of events: RF pulses, gradient applications and collection of data required to produce a MR image.
Quench	The accidental or emergency de-energising of a superconducting magnet by raising the temperature of its cryogen and restoring resistivity.
Readout gradient	Another name for the frequency encoding gradient.
Relaxation	A reduction in strength of the NMV.
Resonance	The transfer of energy from one oscillating object to another having the same frequency of oscillation.
Rise time	The time a gradient coil takes to reach maximum steepness.
RF	Radiofrequency.
RF amplifier	The component of the MRI system which provides energy to the RF transmitter coil.
RF pulse	A short, measured application of RF energy via the RF transmitter coil.
Shielding	Methods used to prevent fringe fields.
Shimming	Passing current through additional 'shim' coils to improve the homgeneity of the main magnetic field of a MR system.
Short time (or Tau) inversion recovery	STIR. A useful sequence for eliminating signal from fat.
Signal to noise ratio	SNR. The ratio of useful MR signal to background signal or 'noise'.
Specific absorption rate (SAR)	A measure of the amount of energy deposited in tissue by radiofrequency waves. Measured in watts per kilogram (W/kg).
Spin echo	An echo resulting from the application of a 180° refocusing pulse.
T1 time	Is the time taken for 63% of longitudinal magnetisation of a tissue to recover.
T2 time	Is the time taken for 63% of the transverse magnetisation of a tissue to decay.

TE	Echo time
Tesla	A unit of measurement of magnetic field strength.
TI	Inversion time.
TR	Repetition time.
Turbo factor	The number of phase encoding steps acquired per TR in fast spin echo imaging. Also known as 'echo train length'.
Turbo spin echo	TSE. A fast imaging sequence, also referred to by some manufacturers as fast spin echo (FSE).
Voxel	Three-dimensional picture element (pixel × slice thickness).
Wave guide	A narrow opening in the scan room wall which allows cables, tubing etc. to enter the room whilst maintaining the integrity of the Faraday cage.
Weighting	Refers to the predominant influence on image contrast of a particular sequnce: T1, T2, PD etc.
Window level	The user-defined level of brightness of the shades of grey viewed in an image.
Window width	The user-definable range of shades of grey included in the viewed image.
Zipper	Common name given to the artefact produced by stray radiofrequency produced within the scan room or 'leaking' in through the Faraday cage.

GLOSSARY

Index